Praise for *The Anti-Estrogenic Diet*

"I strongly support *The Anti-Estrogenic Diet,* which provides simple guidelines for how to reach an optimal hormonal balance that revitalizes and protects the organism."

—DANIEL KUHN, MD, founder of
Integrative Neural Psychiatric Services of New York

"*The Anti-Estrogenic Diet* is a must-read for anyone who cares about their own health, the health of their family, and the health of our global economy."

—SCOTT TREADWAY, PhD, world-renowned botanical expert and
assistant director of Naturally Occurring Standard Group

Praise for *The Warrior Diet*

"We're so convinced that we've found 2002's 25 best (the fastest, easiest, cheapest, and most effective) get-fit solutions, that we are awarding them a prize ... FIRST'S first annual Slimmys for weight-loss excellence. When it comes to diets, we weed the godsends from the gimmicks and give you the very best every issue. But our pick for best of the best? The Slimmy goes to ... *The Warrior Diet.*"

—*First For Women* magazine

"Women everywhere are raving about the super-effective 'warrior' diet—eating lightly during the day, feasting after dark, and losing weight at record speeds."

—*Woman's World,* November 2002

"Rare in books about food, there is wisdom in the pages of *The Warrior Diet* ... Ori Hofmekler knows the techniques, but he shows you a possibility—a platform for living your life as well. *The Warrior Diet* is a book that talks to all of you—the whole person hidden inside."

—UDO ERASMUS, author of *Fats That Heal, Fats That Kill*

OTHER BOOKS BY ORI HOFMEKLER

The Anti-Estrogenic Diet

The Warrior Diet

MAXIMUM
MUSCLE
MINIMUM
FAT

THE SECRET SCIENCE BEHIND
PHYSICAL TRANSFORMATION

ORI HOFMEKLER

Foreword by Marty Gallagher

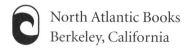

North Atlantic Books
Berkeley, California

Published by
North Atlantic Books
P.O. Box 12327
Berkeley, California 94712

Cover and book design by Suzanne Albertson
Printed in the United States of America

Maximum Muscle, Minimum Fat: The Secret Science Behind Physical Transformation is sponsored by the Society for the Study of Native Arts and Sciences, a nonprofit educational corporation whose goals are to develop an educational and cross-cultural perspective linking various scientific, social, and artistic fields; to nurture a holistic view of arts, sciences, humanities, and healing; and to publish and distribute literature on the relationship of mind, body, and nature.

North Atlantic Books' publications are available through most bookstores. For further information, call 800-733-3000 or visit our website at www.northatlanticbooks.com.

MEDICAL DISCLAIMER: The following information is intended for general information purposes only. Individuals should always see their health care provider before administering any suggestions made in this book. Any application of the material set forth in the following pages is at the reader's discretion and is his or her sole responsibility.

Library of Congress Cataloging-in-Publication Data

Hofmekler, Ori, 1952–
      Maximum muscle and minimum fat : the secret science behind physical transformation / by Ori Hofmekler.
            p. cm.
      "Originally published in 2003 by Dragon Door Publications."
      Summary: "Maximum Muscle Minimum Fat challenges common diet and fitness concepts. Cutting through the confusion of claims, speculations, and pseudo-science often associated with modern diets, fitness, and bodybuilding, the book reveals the true fundamental biological principles of muscle gain and fat loss"—Provided by publisher.
      ISBN 978-1-55643-689-5
      1. Physical fitness. 2. Weight loss. 3. Bodybuilding—Physiological aspects. 4. Nutrition. 5. Metabolism. I. Title.
      RA781.H617 2005
      613.7—dc22   2007047470
                                                                                                       CIP

2 3 4 5 6 7 8 9 Versa 14 13 12 11 10 09 08

CONTENTS

PART I
The Biological Switches That Trigger
Muscle Gain and Fat Loss 1

PART II
Muscle Gain 21

Part III
Fat Loss 101

Part IV
Muscle Gain and Fat Loss Conclusions 123

FOREWORD

Ori Hofmekler: Iconoclastic Innovator

We live in an age of fraudulent fitness. In a society plagued by obesity, impotency, sterility, cardiovascular disorder, and cancer, the public *demands* miracle products, pills, and potions that will fix any and all health and fitness related problems—and fix them instantly. Fitness frauds and charlatans are only too happy to supply the public the miracle products they demand. The biggest myth in all of fitness is that magical products exist that can build muscle and melt off body fat with the greatest of ease. In the old Soviet Union the workers had a saying, "We pretend to work and they pretend to pay us." This slogan could be modified for modern fitness: "We provide pretend products to aide the public in their pretend fitness efforts." Fitness myths perpetuated by fitness frauds have one purpose and one purpose only: to entice members of the fitness community to spend large chunks of their disposable income purchasing bogus products. Anytime a "fitness expert" tells you that building muscle or shedding fat can be made easy, be aware that you are being manipulated into making a purchase. The fitness product pushers produce products that promise exactly what the gullible public wants to hear: By buying "breakthrough" products you will magically be able to eliminate all the toil, tears, teeth-grinding effort, and tough work required to trigger a true transformation.

Ori Hofmekler is the polar opposite of the modern fitness product pusher. He is a fitness heretic, an iconoclastic innovator, a man rooted in science and biology who tells his readers the inconvenient truth about renovating the human body: true transformation is difficult and demanding. What, on an elemental level, defines real physical transformation? If you boil it down to an irreducible core, the savvy fitness adherent would discover that true transformation is about building muscle and melting off body fat. Building muscle is hard work. Shedding body fat is hard work. That's the factual truth. That's the bad news. The good news is that Ori Hofmekler reveals to readers of *Maximum Muscle, Minimum Fat* heretofore-secret science and legitimate, proven methods that can and will build muscle and melt off excess body fat. His nutrition and training systems are grounded in survival science, human biology, and physiology. His methods and tactics are unlike anything you have ever encountered. His methodology is twofold: first he educates the reader with hard science (the physiological science alone makes this book an indispensable reference source), then he provides groundbreaking training protocols. His studied usage of regular food, the kind purchased from the grocery store, is both sane and effective. His approach toward training is both sane and effective. If you are serious about building muscle and melting off body fat, the information contained in this book will provide you with the perfect game plan—*the* tactical approach you need to turn fitness dreams and desires into concrete reality.

I am quite convinced that the Hofmekler template is revolutionary. His strategic approach toward training and nutrition are totally unlike any system I have encountered in my forty-plus years of complete immersion in the health and fitness culture. His nutritional strategies are certainly the most radical and heretical approach to the studied use of food I have ever been exposed to. He is, I am convinced, the ultimate authority on renovating the human body through the use of food and exercise. This book is nothing less than a call to action for those serious about attaining "maximum muscle, minimum fat."

—MARTY GALLAGHER, Olympic lifting and powerlifting champion;
national and world championship team coach; columnist for
The WashingtonPost.com; and author of *The Purposeful Primitive*

January 2008

INTRODUCTION

A Revolutionary Way of Looking at
Maximum Muscle and Minimum Fat

The Renaissance culture that flourished in fifteenth- and sixteenth-century Italy idealized the classic muscular body, promoted in part by Michelangelo and Leonardo da Vinci. These two great artists attempted to define the ideal human body proportions through drawing and sculpture. The last sixty years, however, have brought dramatic changes in the way men and women treat their bodies. We are now living in a seemingly new renaissance of "body adoration," and more people than ever are dieting and exercising, striving to build bodies that are hard and lean.

The goal of achieving a lean and muscular body began long before the time of da Vinci and Michelangelo. The admiration of muscularity and physical power was depicted in ancient Assyrian, Philistine, Minoic, Greek, and Roman art. Physical power was perceived as a primal male virtue required for protecting one's family and defeating or dominating other males.

According to anthropologist Desmond Morris,[1] women are attracted to hard and muscular men with the potential to become strong mates and protectors of their children. But nowadays, women's desire to look hard and lean is almost as great as men's. Without delving more deeply into the anthropological definition of "lean 'n' mean," the question is: Why do you want to build muscle and lose fat? The most obvious answers are that a hard and lean body:

- Is attractive
- Is healthy
- Earns admiration

Many people, and perhaps most, want to gain muscle and lose fat primarily because they believe that a muscular and lean body looks great. Although that is certainly true, there is a great deal of confusion as to how muscular and lean the body should be. For many men and women, looks come first, whereas health and performance come second. Nothing is wrong with a passionate desire to look big and lean. But big muscles do not guarantee maximum power, and a lean look isn't always a sign of health, especially in women. In spite of dieting and exercising more than ever, people today are getting fatter and sicker than ever. The vast majority of modern fitness enthusiasts are failing to improve their conditioning in spite of following steady exercise routines.

The purpose of this book is to cut through the confusion of claims, speculations, and pseudo-science often associated with modern diets and fitness programs, and to present the hard-core truths about muscle gain and fat loss. Based on science and epidemiological evidence, the book offers a revolutionary way of improving human conditioning and performance. Science is about predictions based on predictable fact. Life is about surprises based on the unpredictable reality. This book is about both.

PART I

The Biological Switches
That Trigger Muscle Gain
and Fat Loss

CHAPTER 1

Turning On the Anabolic Switch

C an you turn on your anabolic switch like you can flip on a light? Can you really break the body's secret code to build muscle? For that matter, is there truly a secret code to building muscle? The answer to all these questions is a short and simple *yes!* There is indeed an anabolic switch that can be turned on when the body is in a survival mode. As you're about to read, the anabolic switch that stimulates muscular development is installed within you. All you need to do is acquire the knowledge of how to turn it on. What you're about to read here is revolutionary and may very well go against anything you've known before. But take this information any way you wish. In truth, it simply works.

There is plenty of confusion today about the meaning of *anabolism* and *catabolism.* Bodybuilders commonly believe that *anabolic* means good and *catabolic* means bad. But nothing is further from the truth. To understand what really puts the body into a maximum anabolic potential to rejuvenate tissues and build muscle, first let's briefly shed some light on the anabolic and catabolic forces that regulate our lives.

Anabolism and Catabolism

Your life, biologically speaking, is defined by your metabolism. The process of turning matter into energy and energy back into matter is what makes a living creature superior to any mechanical machine. Your body is programmed to recreate itself every minute of your life. Substances in the form of air, food, water, carbon dioxide, and waste are constantly moving in and out of your body. The process by which material is built is called anabolism, and the process by which material is broken down and removed from the body is called catabolism. It is the balance between the anabolic and catabolic forces that regulate your body fat, muscle mass, rate of aging, and overall health. Both anabolism and catabolism are critical to your survival and, as you'll learn shortly, the two processes work together, activating and potentiating each other.

Negative-Feedback Control

Like many other forces that are necessary to sustain life, anabolic and catabolic processes are naturally regulated in your body through negative-feedback mechanisms, a most efficient form of biological control that regulates the balance between two opposing forces. Many if not most of the body's life functions—such as the regulation of blood sugar, stabilization of blood pressure, assimilation of nutrients, and the stimulation of hormone synthesis—are based on a negative-feedback control.

Most life processes occur in cycles. The body maintains its homeostasis (optimum, balanced metabolic environment) through a negative-feedback control system that cycles continually among antagonistic forces that influence our capacity to survive. The anabolic and catabolic processes regulate each other through these numerous negative-feedback loops. Hormone levels, cellular energy levels, and overall nutritional states are all factors that dictate whether your body builds and repairs tissue or destroys, recycles, burns, or removes material. Simply stated, according to the body's negative-feedback control:

Anabolism is stimulated by catabolic activity.
Catabolism is stimulated by anabolic activity.

For instance, resistance training is actually a catabolic activity that tears muscle fibers, and this catabolic activity triggers an anabolic process by which the body repairs and builds stronger muscle that can handle more stress. For that matter, a novice trainee who has just started lifting weights will most likely experience fast gain in muscularity and strength.

Interestingly, just the opposite may occur when a person maximizes his or her anabolic potential. Trained bodybuilders and powerlifters who have achieved peak muscular development are the ones most likely to face the risk of muscle waste or reach a stagnation point after which they fail to gain more muscle mass or strength. Those active individuals who experience muscle loss surprisingly gain it all back due to the so-called "muscle memory." It seems clear that the body has its own muscle mass set point. It will try to sustain this set point by regulating muscle gain or muscle loss accordingly. People often feel that they are getting weaker in spite of adhering to a diet and exercise routine. What they don't realize is that at a peak anabolic state, the body's catabolic activity increases as if it is trying to shrink the body down to its normal size. Nevertheless, in spite of the above limitations, it is still possible to break plateaus, grind limits, and activate a most powerful anabolic state. How? By following a special dietary cycle that methodically induces a temporary catabolic state, which will then stimulate an anabolic potential that if materialized properly will prohibit the body from reaching a stagnation point. Let's examine how this approach works.

How to Materialize Maximum Growth Potential

To maximize growth, you must activate the hormones that stimulate growth. Hormonal stimulation is actually the switch that turns on the anabolic process, and this very switch gets flipped whenever you fast or undereat. That may go against anything you've heard before, but regardless, here are the facts. Fasting or undereating sends a starvation-like signal that is perceived by the body as catabolic. To compensate for the missing food and to protect itself from metabolic breakdown, the body will boost its anabolic activities, spontaneously increasing its capacity to assimilate protein and other nutrients in order to ensure maximum nutrient utilization from minimum food. It also conserves muscle tissue by inhibiting protein breakdown.

At the cellular level, a most powerful factor is activated during fasting or undereating. This cellular factor is a by-product of energy metabolism and it activates anabolic-stimulating hormones that are secreted by the region of the brain called the hypothalamus and by the pituitary gland, the latter a pea-sized structure located at the base of the brain. Additionally, there is evidence of a dramatic increase in insulin-like growth factor 1 (IGF1) receptors in muscle cell membranes during fasting or undereating. This increase is probably a primal biological compensation mechanism that ensures human survival during periods of limited accessibility to food. In fact, studies on growth hormone reveal a positive correlation between hunger and stimulation of this tissue-building hormone.

Ancient people cycled between periods of undereating, when food was scarce, and periods of overeating, when food was abundant. Over eons of evolution, the human body had been well adapted to withstand periods of undereating. When you undereat, you trigger a primal biological mechanism that helps your body adapt to food deprivation and better survive in times of hardship.

Given all the above, the duration of undereating must be controlled. To take full advantage of this powerful dietary cycle and to avoid metabolic decline and muscle breakdown, you should always fully control the length of undereating, which should never exceed more than twenty-four hours. Also, the incorporation of special recovery meals after exercise will further enhance the overall anabolic impact on the muscles. More on this topic in upcoming chapters.

How to Turn Growth Potential into Muscle Gain

Undereating, overeating, and exercise all force your body to activate and reactivate anabolic states in which the body is pushed to break, repair, build, rejuvenate, and improve itself. During undereating and exercise, the body triggers an anabolic potential that will turn into actual repair and growth of muscle tissues after nutritional replenishment and while the body is in a state of rest. Cycles of undereating and overeating can last from one day per week to continuously, seven days per week. Another bonus of this method is that it forces the body to detoxify. Liver detoxification is critical for the proper production of steroid hormones and the proper utilization of food for energy and growth. Other benefits of detox are the recycling of broken cells and proteins for overall rejuvenation of tissues.

Undereating

Undereating on a daily basis should last up to twenty hours followed by four hours of nourishment from a main meal. During this time, individuals consume fewer calories than they expend (negative energy balance). This means that undereating lasts from one nightly meal to the next nightly meal. However, biologically the body most likely shifts into an actual undereating phase only in the morning hours, after completion of the digestion process.

"Undereating" is a relative term. What is considered undereating for some people may be considered overeating for others. For undereating to have its maximum effect on your body, regulate the amount of food and the length of undereating period based on your specific needs.

According to Dr. Mark Mattson, Chief of the Laboratory of Neurosciences at the National Institute on Aging in Baltimore, Maryland, studies on mice revealed that feeding cycles of fasting one day followed by overeating the next day have shown to be effective enough to help improve survival capabilities such as resistance to stress, protection against insulin resistance, improved brain vitality, and increased life span. In an article on the effect of meal frequency on health,[2] Dr. Mattson expresses his view about the benefits of following an eating cycle based on one main meal per day.

As for the practical applications of undereating, as noted previously it's important for physically active individuals to incorporate small recovery meals during the undereating phase to take advantage of this awesome anabolic potential to assimilate nutrients and protein in the muscle, particularly after exercise.

When incorporating the above feeding cycle, use common sense. If you wish to practice undereating as part of your daily routine, the principle is very simple: Eat one main meal a day, preferably at night. Use your instinct rather than obsessively count hours, calories, or macronutrients.

Those who wish to incorporate undereating for longer than one day should simply try to maintain a negative energy balance in which more energy is expended than consumed. Nonetheless, chronic undereating may lead to a metabolic shutdown; therefore keeping to the cycle of undereating and overeating (rather than chronic undereating) is a must. If you undereat for a couple of days, try to compensate and overeat the following day, preferably during your main evening meal. In any case, it is important to maintain full daily nourishment—including all essential nutrients and sufficient amounts of protein—to avoid muscle waste and overall metabolic decline.

Exercise on an Empty Stomach

Exercising on an empty stomach before you have eaten a meal is a most effective way to maximize the stimulation of an anabolic state while forcing the body to burn fat and inhibit fat gain. People who exercise first thing in the morning or at any other time on an empty stomach are putting themselves in a win-win situation, maximizing the anabolic potential while accelerating the breakdown of fat for energy. As noted, to take advantage of the impact of exercising on an empty stomach, you should have a recovery meal following the workout that supplies all the right nutrients needed for the materialization of repair and growth.

What to Eat During the Undereating Phase

For the purpose of activating growth potential, *undereating* means minimizing your food consumption to mainly low-glycemic fruits and vegetables or their juices, as well as small servings of light fresh protein such as yogurt, poached or boiled eggs, or an all-natural low-glycemic protein shake or a bar made with quality whey.

While undereating, you can have coffee, tea, or unsweetened hot chocolate. However, to avoid an insulin spike that might inhibit the activation of desirable growth-stimulating cellular factors, at no time during this phase should you eat processed carbohydrates or sugar. To be effective, the actual undereating phase should last from wake-up until the evening meal. If once in a while you are in a situation with limited accessibility to food and you're forced to fast or undereat for a whole day (or eat a single meal earlier in the day), that's OK. Nonetheless, to avoid metabolic decline and muscle waste, you should try to limit the duration of undereating to twenty-four hours. As noted previously, if you exercise during the day, you should have a recovery meal after each workout to inhibit protein breakdown and materialize the anabolic activity in the worked muscles. (See the section entitled "Post-Exercise Recovery Meals" in Chapter 8.)

Overeating

Like undereating, *overeating* is a relative term. What one person considers overeating may be normal eating to another. What overeating really means is eating more than you usually do. Regardless of how much you eat, you should always choose whole foods from all the food groups: proteins, fats, and carbohydrates.

Start with protein and veggies, the nutrients your body needs most, and then add fuel foods—the carbs or fat. Make sure you eat whole and complete protein foods such as eggs, fish, dairy, meat, or vegetarian combinations such as grains and beans in order to supply your body with all the essential amino acids.

Include in your daily dietary regimen essential oils such as flaxseed, hempseed, or fish oils that are rich in omega-3 fatty acids. Omega-6 oils do not need to be added or supplemented, as they are abundantly found in the food that we commonly eat. Omega-3 oils are often deficient and must be added or supplemented. Essential fatty acids (EFAs) are critical for all life functions, including brain development, cell membrane formation, and prostaglandin and hormone synthesis. Periodic overeating signals the body to accelerate its metabolic rate to burn all those mega-calories. Over time, periodic cycles of undereating and overeating will most likely help boost your metabolism so you'll be able to eat even more food and thus further accelerate muscle nourishment without worrying about gaining fat.

The Great Pump—A Day After Competition

Professional bodybuilders know about "the Great Pump" they often get the day after a competition.

The term "muscle pump" means a post-exercise swelling of muscles and veins that gives the body a full, muscular, and more plump look.

A competitive bodybuilder who goes through a grueling calorie—or carb-restrictive diet before competition is knowingly ready to sacrifice muscle mass to look lean and defined on stage. But to his surprise, it is the day after the competition when he really looks his best, unfortunately too late to score. The reason is that during a low-calorie, low-carb, pre-competition diet, the body actually goes through a prolonged (chronic-like) undereating phase, which, unlike a short-term undereating phase, is often catabolic—causing a loss of muscle mass and strength.

As noted, during the undereating phase, the body is being stimulated to activate a growth potential that in this case will finally be materialized right after the competition, when the competitive bodybuilder allows himself to eat to his heart's content. It is the pre- and post-competition cycle (i.e., undereating followed by overeating) that forces the body to reach a maximum anabolic state, and that's exactly what happens the day after competition. Experienced and educated bodybuilders know this, and some do a light carb-loading before competing to avoid looking flat and to get maximum muscle pump.

Feeding Cycle

Example of Daily Undereating

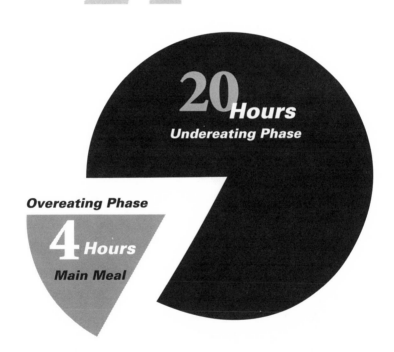

Memory Aid: "**Hours in a Day**" 24

20 **Hours**
Undereating Phase

Overeating Phase
4 **Hours**
Main Meal

CHAPTER 2

Muscle Gain and Fat Loss
at the Cellular Level

To gain muscle and lose fat effectively, you need to understand the basic principles of growth and fat-burning. The most basic, self-contained unit of life in your body is the cell, where every life action begins. Both growth and fat-burning depend on the body's ability to activate certain compounds called cellular factors or cellular messengers, which promote protein synthesis or fat breakdown. A nearly endless number of cellular and systemic events are required for the repair, synthesis, and buildup of muscle tissues, as well as the breakdown of adipose (fat) tissues, thereby turning fat into energy.

Cyclic AMP

If someone told you about a miracle pill that stimulates the body to build muscle and burn fat, you might think it sounds too good to be true. What if you learned that your body already has this miracle pill built in? Your body is preprogrammed with an inner mechanism that, once activated, can stimulate growth potential while simultaneously burning fat. This mechanism works in a way that may contradict much of the information you get from fitness and muscle magazines, but— no surprise—the truth may be too sophisticated for these magazines and, most importantly, it is "anti-industry." For fitness and muscle magazines, advertisements always, always come first, and the truth often comes nowhere near. Here are the facts.

When you fast, exercise, or undergo intense stress, you activate an inner cellular process that induces the synthesis of growth-stimulating hormones while forcing the body to dig into its storage cells and turn glycogen and fat into energy. As if this weren't enough, the same process simultaneously inhibits fat gain. The mechanism that regulates these actions is triggered by a cellular factor, a nucleotide called cyclic adenosine monophosphate (cAMP).

Cyclic AMP's growth-stimulating impact isn't a simple feature. Let's examine how cAMP generates its anabolic stimulating and fat-burning actions. When activated, cAMP catalyzes a chain of cellular events that triggers enzymes responsible for protein synthesis and energy production. A cascade of phosphorylation events (i.e., the addition of phosphorus to enzymes) amplifies the actions of cAMP, including the breakdown of glycogen stores in the liver and muscle and the induction of lipolysis (fat-burning) in fat cells. cAMP also promotes events associated with growth functions—in particular, the release of hormones that stimulate the synthesis of anabolic hormones such as human growth hormone and steroid male hormones.

The Biological Benefits of Stress and Hunger

There is a biological correlation between hunger, stress, and survival. It is now known that hunger, danger, and physical stress trigger a survival mechanism in which cellular levels of cAMP increase, thereby increasing energy production and fat-burning while inducing growth stimulation. cAMP functions to help improve reactions to stress, increasing energy production and overall endurance, all of which are critical for sustaining life. Simply said, cAMP helps support human survival during times of extreme conditions involving physical and nutritional stress. A threshold time is needed for activation of this cellular process, and the time depends on variables such as nutritional state and intensity of stress applied (undereating or exercise). Undereating combined with exercise likely shortens the threshold time needed to turn cAMP into a dominant factor in the cell. Cyclic AMP is promoted by the stress and fat-burning hormones adrenaline and glucagon. The following information may seem a bit technical but is nevertheless important for understanding the workings of this awesome mechanism that forces the body to burn fat and stimulates muscular development.

The adrenal hormones stimulate an enzyme called adenylate cyclase to synthesize cAMP from the energy molecule ATP. Undereating or exercising that often induces a feeling of hunger and stress puts the body in fight-or-flight mode. In this survival mode, the adrenal and glucagon hormones activate compounds called G proteins, which increase cellular levels of cAMP.

G proteins are involved in critical life processes. They mediate numerous functions including the sensations of taste and smell, light detection, and the growth of nerves. Humans and other animals have an inherent increased capacity to sense things when hungry. This enhanced ability to sense the environment most likely helped species hunt, fight, or flee if needed, thus enhancing survival. And the mechanism that triggers this sensual wiring is regulated by G proteins and their related cAMP.

The entire process by which cAMP is synthesized—from the first step of hormonal binding to the final activation of cAMP—is critical for the regulation of basic reactions to stress. cAMP helps improve overall survival capabilities through wiring the senses, increasing alertness, stimulating tissue repair, and improving energy utilization by turning glycogen and fat storage to energy.

Eating full meals inhibits cAMP. Evidently, most modern diets do not sufficiently stimulate the production of cAMP. This fat-burning, growth-stimulating agent is all but suppressed in our modern lifestyle, chronically inhibited by poor eating habits that typically involve consuming too many meals or ingesting too many carbohydrates during the day. Inhibited cAMP could very well be a major reason for the current epidemic of obesity, weight gain, stubborn fat gain, diabetes, and diseases related to premature aging.

Can You Gain Muscle Without Gaining Fat?

Whether or not a person can gain muscle mass without gaining fat is a controversial question. The prospect of gaining muscle mass without gaining fat seems too good to be true. Professional athletes, including boxers, martial artists, and bodybuilders, often fluctuate between twenty and fifty pounds of weight on- and off-season. Off-season, they desperately try to gain weight (muscle and fat), while on-season they try to shed excess body fat to ideally achieve lean muscle gains. However, there are down sides to this method. First, gaining fat during the off-season may cause the formation of stubborn fat tissue. Thus, it may become increasingly difficult in future seasons to lose fat and reach maximum definition. Second, the on-season, which consists of about four to six months of a reduced-calorie, low-carb diet, may adversely affect thyroid hormone functions and slow the basal metabolic rate.

Some athletes are aware of these on- and off-season diet-related setbacks, so they try to avoid significant weight fluctuations by staying lean all year round.

Nevertheless, the notion of gaining muscle, with the inevitable consequence of gaining fat, is still deeply rooted, and rightly so. Under normal dietary routines that involve many meals throughout the day, gaining the undesirable fat while gaining muscle is indeed inevitable. Conventional diets that incorporate long periods of off-season overfeeding and long periods of on-season undereating are probably missing the opportunity to take advantage of the biological principles upon which the body can potentially build muscle while losing fat.

cAMP is a critical element in stimulating a growth potential. Nonetheless, for the materialization of this growth potential, another cellular factor must be activated—one responsible for the translation of the growth potential into actual muscle gain. Without its finalizing actions, there will be no tissue repair or growth. Here is how this cellular factor works. When eating a full meal right after fasting or exercising (protein, carbs, fat), you actually trigger an inner mechanism that helps your body recuperate from induced stress. Your body gains an increased capacity to replenish energy reserves and nourish starving tissue with lost nutrients. It also gains the actual capacity to build and repair damaged tissues. All these actions are regulated by a cellular factor called cyclic guanine monophosphate (cGMP). cGMP is insulin-dependent and is therefore instantly activated when eating carbohydrate meals. cGMP appears to inhibit the actions of cAMP by counteracting cAMP's effects. Nonetheless, under normal conditions these two cellular factors work in sync, balancing each other through a negative-feedback control; one is a stimulator whereas the other is an activator. One starts the process and the other finalizes it, and so forth.

Partitioning: Converting Fat to Muscle

The human body is not built efficiently enough to go through long periods of induced overfeeding or induced underfeeding without adverse side effects. On the other hand, short periods of controlled undereating and overeating are likely to activate the cellular forces that help make possible simultaneous muscle gain and fat loss. In fact, some powerful anabolic agents (such as growth hormone) deliver their action by diverting fat fuel energy into protein synthesis. This process of using fat energy to build muscle is called "partitioning."

cGMP: Enhancing Thyroid Actions

Though not a steroid, the thyroid hormone has a steroid-like activity. It plays a critical role in regulating energy production, body heat, steroid hormone activity, and fat-burning. cGMP maximizes thyroid hormone utilization. To be fully effective, the thyroid hormone must be converted from T4 into its most active form, T3. This conversion from T4 to T3 is catalyzed by a high level of cellular ATP that signals the body that "plenty of energy is available." cGMP, which is activated by high cellular energy, signals the thyroid to accelerate its actions and thus boost the body's metabolic rate.

One of the main reasons for a metabolic decline is an inactive thyroid. The thyroid hormone can deactivate itself by reversing its active T3 form into a reverse T3 (rT3), an inactive form. Reverse T3 is formed when not enough cellular energy is available over a prolonged period of time, a situation that may be due to over-restrictive low-calorie or low-carb diets. This reverses the order of the rings in the iodine atoms in the thyroid hormone molecule and creates a mirror-like image of T3 (which is why it's called reverse T3). rT3 is not easily detected by a routine blood test. Nevertheless, its potentially adverse effect on muscle gain, fat loss, and overall metabolism can be devastating.

People who go through long periods of crash or low-carb diets often suffer from impaired thyroid function, with symptoms such as sensitivity to cold (especially cold hands), low body temperature, dry skin, loss of hair, sluggish metabolism, and overall fatigue. When properly activated in the body's machinery, cGMP helps optimize thyroid functions, ensuring optimum energy utilization for all life functions and sustaining a healthy metabolism.

cGMP and Potency

cGMP might be regarded as a sex-stimulating cellular factor. In fact, the drug Viagra works on the principle of inhibiting cellular cGMP reuptake. cGMP, with its insulin-related actions, promotes the production of nitric oxide (NO). NO, a metabolite of the amino acid arginine, is a natural compound that regulates blood pressure and circulation. As a vasodilator, NO is critical for male erection as well as female sexual arousal. NO and cGMP are responsible for the unrestricted flow of blood into the erectile chamber of the penis. It is cGMP that helps induce a high level of local NO production.

Sexual arousal is a unique event in which both cGMP and cAMP are activated simultaneously. While cGMP dilates the blood vessels to ensure proper blood flow, cAMP constricts blood vessels to trap the blood in the erectile chamber, which helps maintain a full, steady, stiff erection. The activation of the enzyme phosphorylase diesterase (PDE), which deactivates cAMP, ends an erection, thus allowing the blood to flow out of the erectile chamber.

Overall, cGMP is critical for potency and virility. Men and women who chronically undereat may be able to live longer but may risk living life with a diminished libido.

Chronic Elevation of cGMP

Chronic domination of any cellular factor can be detrimental to your health. Chronic elevation of cellular cGMP, caused by eating too many meals or by frequently ingesting carbohydrates during the day, will chronically inhibit cAMP and counteract its biological benefits. Under cGMP regulatory actions, enzymes that break glycogen and fat stores are inactivated, and thus under such conditions cGMP will inhibit fat-burning while enhancing fat deposits.

Chronic elevation of cGMP upsets the body's biological balance; more material (i.e., fat and toxins) is deposited than removed. The inability to detoxify compromises liver functions, further accelerating the accumulation of metabolic waste toxins and fat in body tissue. This adverse process often results in excessive weight gain, sluggish metabolism, insulin resistance, lack of energy (with cravings for sweets), general fatigue, and accelerated aging.

The Combustion Engine Principle
Or, The Pistons that Drive the Body's Machinery

The body's metabolism operates in a similar way to that of a combustion engine. The constant shift between antagonistic cellular forces activates and deactivates body chemistry that moves the metabolic pistons up and down, like those of a combustion engine in motion. The cycling between cellular factors cAMP and cGMP is the principal factor that moves and drives the metabolic wheels that generate energy. cAMP and cGMP polarize the direction in which cellular actions occur. This polarization is crucial for the integrity of all evolving metabolic actions, from burning matter into energy, to depositing material and replenishing energy.

Like a combustion engine based on the principle of high and low pressure, your biological engine is based on opposing forces that move your metabolic pistons. When one piston is up, the other piston is down. Cycling between these cellular forces (such as through undereating and overeating) puts the spin on your charging wheels.

Any action you perform chronically may offset your biological engine. Chronic activation of one cellular factor chronically deactivates its opposing factor. As noted, most current diets chronically deactivate cAMP while chronically inducing cGMP. That is why undereating, with its cAMP-related actions, is so critical for the initial charging of your metabolism. cAMP stimulates growth potential while inducing breakdown of fat for energy. Nonetheless, this is only the first step in moving the wheels of the body's machinery. In the next step, this (high-pressure) stress-related cellular factor will spin the metabolic wheel into a lower-pressure insulin-related cellular factor, cGMP. cGMP facilitates growth and replenishes empty energy reserves by building energy stores, thus spinning the metabolic wheel back into cAMP to again break glycogen and fat storage for regenerating energy production while stimulating growth, and so forth. Cyclic AMP and cyclic GMP are cellular factors that, while being cycled, create a combustion-like thrust impact that generates energy and burns fat while facilitating repair, growth, and rejuvenation.

Combustion Engine Principle
Cycling Between cAMP and cGMP

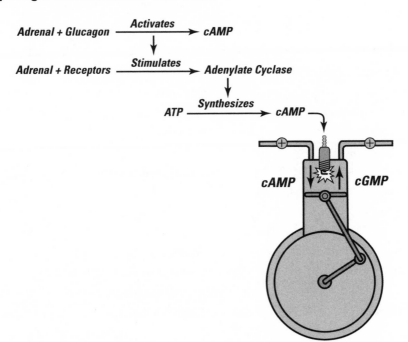

PART II

Muscle Gain

The adoration of the muscular body may well relate to the primal appreciation of human attraction to physical power as a means of survival. For ancient warriors muscularity, strength, and endurance often meant the difference between life and death. In contrast, the modern concept of muscularity has nothing to do with functionality or survival.

The main goal of modern fitness and bodybuilding is to increase muscularity for sheer vanity, whereas performance and health are secondary goals. As a result, the vast majority of people today have been busting their butts to develop a new kind of body, one that hasn't been tested through the evolution of humans. This body image that manifests on the glossy covers of fitness and muscle magazines has nothing to do with biological functions. Not surprisingly, a typical bodybuilder and weekend warrior will fail to perform in a real-life situation that demands high endurance, speed, and agility. In ancient times, the purpose of exercise was to build a powerful body.

Nowadays, the only way to develop a functional powerful body is to drop the modern gimmicks, tricks, and pseudo routines to build muscle mass, and instead step back and start adapting old-fashioned concepts of training. This is not the type of advice you typically read in muscle magazines. The next few chapters discuss the most important biological factors involved in improving body composition for maximized performance. Active individuals will find practical advice on how to apply the information for their specific needs.

Some of the material may seem a bit technical, but it is my wish to present the facts behind the principles of muscle gain and fat loss so as not to disappoint readers who thirst for a full understanding of how the amazing human body works. Also included are clear summaries and conclusions that ideally will make the following information easy to digest.

Growth, including muscle gain, is the outcome of opposing forces and results from an array of biological events that lead to cellular activities such as gene transcription and protein synthesis. Like many other biological functions, growth can either heal or kill. On the positive side, the anabolic process of creating new cells is critical for tissue repair, the replacement of old and dead cells, and the buildup of muscle fibers for improved performance. Growth is a tightly controlled process that facilitates the development of a human being from an early embryonic stage to a fully mature adult.

On the negative side, uncontrolled growth can lead to formation of cancerous tumors and death. Ironically, the most powerful growth stimulants that help keep people young and vigorous could also be the most detrimental to human life under certain circumstances.

Many processes can stimulate growth. However, for every process that induces growth, there is an opposing force that inhibits it. That's how the body protects itself and sustains its homeostasis (metabolic integrity). As noted previously, critical metabolic functions are regulated by negative-feedback mechanisms that are based on a balance between two opposing forces. Interestingly, much of the recent knowledge about growth and its biological regulation in the body is derived from current cancer research.

Most cancer drugs, if not all, act as growth inhibitors. In fact, all anti-inflammatory drugs—including nonsteriodal anti-inflammatory drugs (NSAIDs) such as aspirin or ibuprofen, and blood pressure drugs such as beta blockers—are directly or indirectly suppressors of hormones and enzymes that stimulate growth. When we try to answer the question *What makes a muscle grow naturally without the use of anabolic drugs?*, the answer is anything but simple.

As you'll soon see, the new science of muscle gain is a topic that may seem controversial or even politically incorrect. Substances often considered to be the most adverse to one's health might in fact be the most powerful growth-promoting agents. However, the opposite may also be true: What is regarded as the healthiest and the most beneficial might inhibit growth and even promote fat gain. A wide variety of circumstances and individual constitutions determine the actual outcome.

Even more confusing is the fact that certain anabolic agents might turn out to be catabolic, while some catabolic agents might be extremely anabolic. In the upcoming chapters, we'll cover the most prominent growth-regulating factors, including steroid hormones, fatty acids and their anabolic actions, peptide-stimulating hormones, insulin, growth hormone, growth factors, and also substances and factors that inhibit growth. Finally, understanding the biological principles behind these complex processes will help simplify and clear the picture of what really makes a muscle grow.

Last but not least is the impact of exercise. Exercise can profoundly encourage muscle gain or can retard muscular development and performance. As you'll soon read, proper cycling of exercise, rest, and diet is necessary for maximizing quality muscle gain. Most importantly, special exercises are needed to effectively transform muscle into super muscle tissue with superior strength, speed, and endurance capabilities.

CHAPTER 3

Steroid Hormones: The Most Powerful Growth-Materializing Agents

Steroids are some of the most intriguing of all hormones. Unlike other classes of anabolic or fat-burning hormones, the steroid group exhibits diverse and sometimes contradictory actions. In general, the main function of steroid hormones is to develop and maintain a mature and vigorous body. Some steroids are responsible for stress reactions and regulation of blood sugar; others are responsible for the regulation of minerals. But the most notorious steroids are the sex hormones androgens and estrogens. Androgens are the male sex hormones (including testosterone, its precursors, and its derivatives) and are regarded as the most potent libido enhancers and muscle builders. Nonetheless, it is the balance among all steroid hormones, including the female hormones, stress hormones, and mineralocorticoids, that determines how the body reacts to stress, builds tissue, and sustains life.

Androgens have a long-lasting impact on the body. Their actions can be prolonged for hours or days, making them the most effective anabolic agents. However, as steady and potent as they are, the impact of these anabolic steroids is not as immediate as other hormones such as growth hormone, adrenaline, or insulin. In fact, their impact on the body occurs in a delayed fashion.

Often people can't gain muscle or lose fat because of certain hormonal imbalances or deficiencies. This chapter discusses steroid hormone actions and their practical application to muscle gain and overall health. Let's cover briefly the most important factors necessary for triggering steroid actions.

Steroid Hormone Synthesis

The switch that turns on steroid hormone synthesis is cellular factor cAMP. cAMP and its related enzyme (protein kinase A) induce the release of steroid-stimulating hormones from the pituitary gland. These peptide-stimulating hormones signal the gonads and adrenal glands to synthesize steroid hormones.

Note that steroid hormone synthesis may be inhibited by high levels of circulating cholesterol (even though cholesterol is a necessary precursor to this synthesis). Steroid production depends upon cholesterol synthesis in the mitochondria of cells that manufacture steroid hormones, typically located in the gonad and adrenal glands. High plasma levels of cholesterol have been shown to inhibit cholesterol synthesis.

The conversion of cholesterol (twenty-seven carbon atoms) to steroid hormones involves the rate-limiting cleavage of a six-carbon residue from cholesterol to produce the steroid hormone pregnenolone—"the mother of all steroid hormones," i.e., the precursor for steroid hormones including progesterone, testosterone (and other androgens), estrogen, aldosterone, and cortisol.

Undereating and Exercise Stimulate
Steroid Hormone Synthesis

Steroidal activity can be stimulated by fasting, undereating, and exercise, all of which are cAMP inducers. This may have to do with an inherent, primordial compensating mechanism that has helped humans survive during extreme conditions that involve food deprivation and intense physical stress. Here is how this process works: Lack of food and hunger increase the level of cellular cAMP, which then induces steroid hormone synthesis. The activity of all steroid-producing enzymes (desmolase) is closely affected by this very factor. cAMP catalyzes an enzyme that increases available cholesterol concentration, the substrate to steroid hormone synthesis. cAMP also increases the activity of steroid-producing enzymes by binding to specific genes that increase levels of these enzymes and therefore enhance steroid hormone synthesis.

Peptide-Stimulating Hormones and Their Specific Steroid Hormone Targets

- Luteinizing Hormone (LH)—> Progesterone and Testosterone
- Adrenocorticotropic Hormone (ACTH)—> Cortisol + Adrenal Androgens
- Follicle-Stimulating Hormone (FSH)—> Estradiol
- Angiotensin—> Aldosterone

High Mitochondrial Capacity Required for Proper Steroidal Impact

The mitochondria are energy-producing organelles (with their own DNA) inside the cell, responsible for energy production, particularly from fat. High mitochondrial capacity increases fat utilization and thereby helps promote steroid hormone synthesis. The first critical stage of steroid hormone synthesis involves the conversion of cholesterol into pregnenolone in the mitochondria of steroid-producing cells. The enzyme system that catalyzes the cleavage reactions that lead to steroid hormone synthesis is called desmolase (P-450, SCC).

Mitochondrial damage caused by toxicity, aging, or lack of essential nutrients and antioxidants can lead to lower mitochondrial capacity, which may result in steroid hormone decline, loss of muscle mass, general weakness, and overall metabolic decline. Evidently there is a positive correlation between essential antioxidant and detoxifying nutrients and the capacity to develop a healthy and muscular body.

How Dietary Fat and Cholesterol Affect Steroid Hormones

As noted, cholesterol negatively regulates steroid hormone synthesis. Again, through a negative-feedback control, when cytosolic cholesterol is depleted in steroid-producing cells, cholesterol synthesis is stimulated, and so is its conversion to the steroid hormone pregnenolone, which moves to the cytosol (the intracellular content surrounding the mitochondria) for further processing. Conversely, a high cellular cholesterol level tends to inhibit cholesterol production, thus decreasing steroid hormone synthesis.

Consumption of fats and carbs should then be intelligently manipulated to ensure proper utilization and to prevent insulin resistance as well as over-accumulation of lipids that may impair steroid hormone synthesis and potential muscle gain. Nonetheless, as much as excess of carbs or cholesterol may suppress steroid hormones, so will deficiencies in calories or fat. Prolonged low-fat, low-calorie diets may suppress steroid actions because of a lack of dietary fat, cholesterol, and energy needed for steroid production. In fact, in healthy individuals, high-fat meals can help promote steroid production as long as calorie supply is sufficient.

In times when eating in moderation is considered to be healthiest, it may seem wrong to advise people to overeat. Nevertheless, overeating if done properly can be the most effective way to boost steroidal actions, enhance libido, and maximize growth potential.

High Energy Turnover Enhances Androgen Production

Androgen production depends on the rate of energy production. High energy turnover is a metabolic state that involves high energy intake and high energy expenditure. High energy turnover forces the body to mobilize fat with its cholesterol carrier through the blood to the muscles and liver—where it converts to energy, thus depleting cellular cholesterol levels while enhancing steroid hormone production.

Any exercise method that forces development of muscle with high mitochondrial density will naturally increase the body's capacity to absorb and spend energy. Again, improvement in fat and cholesterol utilization by virtue of improved energy utilization will most likely help sustain peak steroidal activity.

How to Take Advantage of Steroid Hormone Actions

Sex hormones—particularly the male androgens—are considered the most anabolic (tissue-building) hormones. Sex hormones have a profound impact on the body, defining gender, body composition, virility or fecundity, and tissue regeneration. The names "testosterone" and "estrogen" are perhaps the most familiar of hormones among the general population, with the exception of our well-known adrenaline. Nevertheless, there is still much confusion about the biological functions of testosterone and estrogen. It is clear that both hormone levels decline with age, leading to loss of muscle and bone mass, gain and retention of fat, overall metabolic decline, and increased vulnerability to disease.

Males and females produce both hormones. Testosterone, the male hormone, plays a critical role in women's bodies, as does estrogen in men. The female hormone estrogen is necessary for regulation of critical metabolic actions in men's bodies. Sex steroid hormones can convert from one to another. Of special interest to us is the conversion of testosterone into estrogen. This process, discussed later in the chapter, can cause feminization of the male body, including stubborn fat gain, declining testosterone levels, loss of muscle mass, and impaired physical and sexual performance. This very process can devastate the female body as well. When occurring in excess, it can lead to hormonal disorders, undesirable weight gain, and formation of tumors.

Taking advantage of steroid hormone anabolic actions requires more than just an increase in their levels. In fact, too high a level of testosterone may adversely affect its anabolic action. To manipulate anabolic steroid hormones, you should first try to understand how they are regulated in your body.

Regulating Steroid Hormone Levels

The body regulates steroid hormone levels via a tight control mechanism, and any artificial interference with this control mechanism may shatter steroidal anabolic actions.

As noted, the most important anabolic steroid hormones are androgens, including testosterone. The biosynthesis of these hormones is constantly regulated through a tight negative-feedback control. Gonadal-stimulating hormones such as luteinizing hormone (LH) or gonadotropin releasing hormone (GNRH), which are secreted by the pituitary gland and the hypothalamus, respectively, are directly affected by levels of circulating sex hormones.

A high level of androgens inhibits LH secretion, while low levels of androgens signal the hypothalamus to elevate GNRH. This, in turn, increases the pituitary's secretion of LH, a peptide hormone that binds to gonadal tissue and stimulates male sex hormone production.

As you can see, chronic elevation of androgens through drugs or precursor pills (known as "prohormones" openly marketed by the sport nutrition industry) may adversely affect the body's natural hormonal regulation mechanism, eventually shattering its ability to produce these hormones on its own. People who take androgen boosters or drugs without medical supervision should be careful to cycle and monitor the amount and intervals so as to prevent a steroidal decline.

DHT for Maximum Anabolic Impact

The most anabolic steroid hormones are male androgens. Many people suffer from low levels of androgens because of wrong diet, drug abuse, chemical toxicity, overtraining, or aging. Understanding the basic biological processes that involve anabolic steroid production may help protect one from hormonal decline and maintain maximum anabolic impact.

Testosterone is regarded as the most anabolic male steroid hormone. "Big T," however, isn't as big as it seems. In fact, some researchers consider testosterone to be merely a prohormone because of its relatively weak actions compared to other androgens, in particular DHT (dehydrotestosterone).

Testosterone is responsible for many critical functions, the most predominant of which are the defining and developing of male characteristic features, including sexual maturation and fertility. However, testosterone anabolic actions and its related sexual desire and aggression are significantly affected by other androgens, some of which are as potent as testosterone, and even more so. Androgens can typically convert from one form to another, from precursors into hormones. For instance, the adrenal prohormone DHEA can convert to testosterone or estrogen.

Certain enzymes enable other androgens to be converted to testosterone, and further into DHT. DHT is "where the buck stops." It is the most potent male steroid hormone. In fact, its actions are ten times stronger than those induced by testosterone. DHT has been called "bad testosterone" due to its allegedly adverse effect on the prostate. Nevertheless, there is emerging evidence that DHT may not be the real contributing factor to prostate enlargement but rather the female hormone estrogen. When estrogen is present in excess in a male, it has been shown to cause feminization of the body and metabolic disorders including enlargement of the prostate.

Unfortunately, nowadays it is common to prescribe drugs that literally emasculate men. Any medication, drug, or substance that inhibits the conversion of testosterone into DHT (such as prostate and hair loss-related drugs) may also suppress DHT's anabolic actions, thereby adversely affecting libido and sexual performance. In summary, testosterone and DHT play critical roles in growth, potency, and fertility, but when it comes down to muscular development, DHT rules.

How Testosterone and DHT Are Produced

In males, LH binds to leyding cells, which stimulate testosterone production. Testosterone is mobilized to the plasma and also carried to sertoli cells by a special protein carrier—the androgen-binding protein. In sertoli cells, testosterone is converted to DHT. Both T and DHT are carried in the plasma by a specific gonadal steroid-binding globulin (GSBG) until they reach their target. In a number of target tissues, testosterone can convert to DHT.

Aromatizing: The Modern Man's Nightmare

Aromatizing, or the conversion of testosterone to estrogen in the body, is about to become widely considered as one of the most horrific nightmares of modern men. The conversion of testosterone to estrogen via a chemical process called "aromatizing" is a natural occurrence that increases with aging. However, its effects on young adults today are staggering. The enzyme that converts androgens to estrogens, called aromatase, is stimulated by certain industrial chemicals that have similar structure to the female hormone estrogen. These chemicals are commonly found in the food we eat, the water we drink, and the products we use.

To avoid over-expression of the aromatase enzyme, it is important to understand how it works. The aromatase enzyme is responsible for many undesirable estrogen-related actions that cause adverse feminization of men. Aromatase is actually a complex of enzymes (not just one) that is largely produced by adipose (fat) tissue. Normally aromatase plays a critical role in the female body, supporting optimal estrogen levels. In females, luteinizing hormone (LH) binds to cells in the ovary, where it stimulates the synthesis of androstendione and testosterone. Only then does an additional enzyme complex called aromatase finally convert androgens into estrogens.

Certain conditions such as overly high levels of androgens due to steroid drug abuse, a congested liver, or obesity can lead to over-expression of the aromatase enzyme complex, resulting in stubborn fat gain (usually around the belly and chest) and a decline in anabolic androgen level, a condition that eventually inhibits muscle growth. As mentioned previously, aromatase over-activity can also devastate the female body, causing hormonal disorders, disease, and cancer.

Liver detoxification and a reduction in body fat are probably the most beneficial methods for encouraging anti-aromatase activity. Both methods can also help maximize steroid hormone utilization and enhance their anabolic actions. Nonetheless, it is critically important to eliminate aromatase-promoting substances from the diet including pesticides, herbicides, plastic derivatives (particularly from soft, "cloudy" or opaque plastic containers), and estrogenic dietary compounds such as those found in soy, clover, licorice, and hops (in beer). Some anti-aromatase drugs are available, but these have severe and even mortal side effects. The effectiveness of natural anti-aromatase treatments, via herbal or nutritional supplements, is only now gaining a reputation. There is growing evidence that certain compounds in food, herbs, and oils can inhibit aromatase activity. Notable natural sources for anti-aromatase nutrients are garlic, onion, passion flower, chamomile, grass-fed dairy, turmeric, raw nuts and seeds, and omega-3 oils from fish, flaxseed, and hempseed. Additional research is needed for more conclusive evidence of the magnitude and effectiveness of natural therapies compared to drug therapies. (For more on this topic see *The Anti-Estrogenic Diet*, North Atlantic Books, 2007, or log onto www.AntiEstrogenicDiet.com.)

Steroid Promoters vs. Steroid Suppressors

Stimulation of androgen synthesis occurs during fasting and exercise via the activation of cellular factor cAMP and its related actions. High cholesterol levels tend to decrease steroid hormone synthesis. High body fat, excessive level of androgens due to steroid drugs, exposure to estrogenic chemicals, and a stressed liver are all factors that contribute to increased aromatase activity (i.e., increased conversion of testosterone to estrogen), thus adversely affecting testosterone anabolic and sexual impact. Low-fat, low-calorie, and crash diets may suppress steroid hormone levels. High-fat, high-calorie meals may help promote steroidal actions.

The "Cocktail Hormone" Impact

Steroids act together, somewhat like a well-mixed cocktail of hormones. Derived from the gonadals and the adrenal glands, they indirectly enhance or inhibit each other's actions. The adrenal cortex produces three classes of steroid hormones that play important roles in the anabolic process leading to muscle gain.

Some of the adrenal hormones, such as cortisol and aldosterone, are generally considered to be the "bad guys" by bodybuilders and athletes. However, as you'll soon see, there are no good or bad steroids.

In fact, the only "bad guys" are chronically induced substances. When anything occurs chronically, the body loses its own ability to naturally control the complex of forces that keep it alive and well. Each force—whether a cellular factor or an enzyme—regulates or mediates critical life functions. Once chronically inhibited or chronically activated, a biological process that is normally beneficial can lead to a metabolic catastrophe with severe and even mortal consequences.

Take Advantage of the Cortisol Wave

As noted previously, adrenal steroids play a critical role in regulating stress-related reactions, including reactions to physical stress. As you'll see, all adrenal hormones (cortisol, aldosterone, DHEA, etc.) help the body survive in tough, stressful conditions such as physical danger, lack of food, injuries, and the need to endure extreme physical strain.

The three classes of adrenal steroids are glucocorticoids, mineralocorticoids, and androgens:

1. *Glucocorticoids* primarily regulate anti-inflammatory reactions, as well as reactions to shock and hypoglycemia (low blood sugar).
2. *Mineralocorticoids* regulate the body's level of sodium and potassium.
3. *Androgens* regulate the same anabolic and sexual actions as gonadal androgens in males and ovarian-derived androgens in females.

The adrenal cortex consists of three main regions (or zones). Each region produces its own distinct steroid hormones and has its own enzyme balance that, once activated, dictates specific steroid hormone production. Interestingly, the same adrenal zones that produce anabolic androgens can also synthesize the stress hormone cortisol. This fact may relate to a survival mechanism that regulates these two antagonistic forces to prevent the over-expression of each. Biologically, both anabolic androgens and cortisol play important roles in reaction to stress, recuperation, preventing muscle waste, and enhancing tissue repair.

Reach Maximum Anabolic Potential During Exercise

In theory, stress hormones inhibit muscle gain. However, in life, things appear quite differently. In fact, stress and muscle gain go hand in hand, such as during exercise. The level of the stress hormone cortisol rises and falls in a wavelike manner during exercise. Taking advantage of "the cortisol wave" via special exercise intervals may help induce a peak anabolic potential.

This is how it works: Cortisol production is stimulated by the hypothalamic stress-related hormone adrenocorticotropic hormone (ACTH). ACTH is a stimulating hormone that is secreted during stress, exercise, or fasting. It plays a major role in regulating a negative-feedback loop that controls circulating levels of cortisol. Elevated levels of cortisol signal the brain to decrease circulating levels of corticotropin-releasing hormone (the hormone that stimulates ACTH), thus decreasing ACTH and consequently cortisol level as well. That negative-control loop is probably what keeps the cortisol level from skyrocketing during physical stress and gives it a wavelike characteristic.

Both cortisol and androgen levels are elevated during exercise. Nonetheless, the adrenal gland is not a main source of androgen production. In fact, overall androgen levels increase because of an increase in both gonadals and adrenal androgens. For maximum anabolic impact, it's important to keep androgen levels high and cortisol levels low.

Undereating coupled with exercise increases levels of both androgens and cortisol. However, because of the cortisol wave, there is a threshold time by which cortisol levels decrease. This temporary decrease in cortisol level creates a hormonal balance that favors androgen to cortisol and thereby helps increase anabolic potential. Therefore, duration of exercise intervals is most important in defining whether the exercise-related stress will induce an anabolic or a catabolic state. Prolonged and intense exercise routines over forty-five minutes have been shown to lower testosterone levels and thus may be counter-effective. Does it mean that prolonged drills aren't beneficial? Not necessarily. With proper application of recovery meals, one can keep hormones at peak even during prolonged drills.

To take advantage of the cortisol wave, try to incorporate a few minutes of intense pre-workout sets (either resistance exercise or sprint intervals). These pre-workout "shock exercises" will help initiate the cortisol wave, inducing a sharp rise and fall in cortisol levels, providing the body with the environment and the threshold time it needs to maximize anabolic potential for the upcoming workout set.

Supersets and Forced Sets

Supersets and forced sets, if done properly, can help induce a maximum anabolic state. Long resistance supersets that take between one and three minutes followed by a "forced" set (immediately after completion of an intense, pre-exhausting set) will most likely grant the amount of time needed for cortisol levels to rise and fall. This method allows the cortisol level to drop within the time range of the superset and the forced repetition (approximately five minutes). Simply put, relatively long (five to fifteen minutes), grueling, intense sets can increase one's chance of establishing better anabolic potential, as long as the net workout volume doesn't exceed forty-five minutes.

To fully manipulate steroid actions, you should try to take advantage of cortisol waves during exercise. You can do this as follows:

- Keep your workout short (up to forty-five minutes). After intense pre-workout "shock" sets (also called pre-fatigue exercise), do one giant superset, then move on to the next set. Do the same routine again, but without the shock exercise. Continue with your workout in the following way:
- Take short rest intervals between sets (thirty to sixty seconds). Long rests between sets may give the body enough time to snap out of the "action mode" and reset itself to reestablish a high cortisol level during the next set. On the other hand, short rest periods between sets may continue to lower cortisol levels because of the initial elevation of cortisol during the "shock

exercise" (pre-workout set). Again, a high cortisol level marks an upcoming cortisol decline. A low cortisol level marks an upcoming cortisol increase. Therefore, when incorporating short rests between sets the body will gradually adapt to the highly intense drills by shortening cortisol waves and lowering its levels.

Note that, though based on science, this approach needs to be further researched. Nevertheless it makes sense, and most importantly, it works.

As absurd as it may sound, it is the high levels of cortisol that help establish maximum upcoming anabolic potential. In fact, intense training has a profoundly relaxing effect on the body because of the nature of the cortisol wave. For that matter, any exercise can help reduce stress if it is done properly. A physically trained body can cope with stress better than a sedentary one. As noted, through adaptation, the body gets tougher by shortening cortisol spikes and avoiding chronically elevated cortisol levels that are associated with panic reactions and impaired performance.

In summary, adrenal steroids help the body survive under stressful conditions. Manipulating the cortisol wave to work for you means taking advantage of your survival mechanism to get tougher and stronger.

Aldosterone for Survival and Muscle-Toning

Aldosterone is an adrenal mineralocorticoid hormone that regulates ion mineral balance and blood pressure via sodium and potassium pumps. Aldosterone is often regarded as a "bad guy" because of its presumed adverse effects on blood pressure and water retention. It is activated by the hormone angiotensin, derived from the actions of the kidney on the liver.

Aldosterone actions probably helped humans survive during primordial times when salt was not abundant in every community. Salt, once considered a precious commodity, was traded over long distances and even used as currency. (The ancient Greeks regarded salt as a substance that boosts physical power.) Through many years of evolution, the human body has adapted primarily to food that is minimally processed and has a significantly higher ratio of potassium to sodium. Potassium, a natural diuretic mineral, activates aldosterone and also helps remove water from the tissues, thus alleviating edema and water retention.

Looking at how the human body is biologically equipped to better survive under conditions of physical hardship and food deprivation, one might conclude that an inner wisdom is deeply embedded into basic human nature. Physical stress such as exercise, as well as the endurance of periods of lack of food, would likely activate a most powerful inner mechanism that compensates the body for the physical and nutritional stress by inducing metabolic actions that improve the body's capacity to generate energy and resist these stressors. Periodically restricting sodium and eating high-potassium foods would give the body the signal that sodium is scarce and thus trigger this primal survival mechanism that activates the mineralocorticoid aldosterone and its related actions.

There may be yet another bonus involved. Aldosterone, which is responsible for the preservation of sodium, may indirectly help induce a preliminary anabolic potential in which muscle cell membranes are alkalized via sodium pump. When activated, the sodium pump—or as it's also called, the sodium channel—increases sodium ions in the cell, a process necessary for muscle contractions as well as other metabolic functions, including cellular growth.

Aldosterone is a weak steroid, and diets that are overly salty and deficient in potassium chronically deactivate this hormone. Long periods of sodium restriction can reactivate aldosterone but may eventually lead to water retention and elevated blood pressure when sodium is reintroduced. Conversely, loading the body with potassium by eating potassium-rich foods such as avocados, tomatoes, potatoes, and vegetables naturally helps activate aldosterone, staving off undesirable water retention and its related blood-pressure fluctuations. Note that chronic elevation of aldosterone such as with hypertensive individuals is generally a symptom of metabolic disorders that occur due to impaired liver or kidney functions. Bad diets, high levels of toxicity, and lack of exercise are all factors that contribute to impaired capacity of the body to regulate normal metabolic functions, including the homeostasis of minerals.

Aldosterone induces electrical charge in muscle cells by allowing an increase in cellular sodium. This process may help induce muscular action potential with higher overall muscle tone. (Muscle action potential is discussed in more depth in Chapter 8, "Super Muscle.")

Steroid Receptors' Super Actions

The steroid hormone receptors belong to a "superfamily" of proteins that constitute receptors for steroid hormones, thyroid hormones, vitamin D, and vitamin A (retinoic acid). Note that the following may seem technical but it aims to help elucidate the unique nature of the steroid hormones and how these powerful hormones induce their actions. You'll soon realize that unlike other hormones, steroid hormones work directly on genes that regulate critical metabolic functions, including the development of muscle tissues and the breakdown of fat. Also, due to a certain degree of similarity to steroids, some non-steroidal substances such as vitamin A and the thyroid hormone play critical roles in promoting steroid hormone activity.

When activated, steroid hormone receptors bind to specific nucleotide sequences in the DNA, referred to as hormone response elements (HREs). HREs could have either activating or repressing actions on their target genes. Most important, several receptors are included to interact with other transcriptional mediators. For instance, retinoic acid X receptors (RXRs—for vitamin A) have been shown to enhance the DNA binding of thyroid hormone receptors, which have a high affinity for increasing energy production and lowering cholesterol, as well as enhancing steroid hormone synthesis. Vitamin A works as a co-factor in steroidal activity; steroid receptor binding to DNA is the very factor that induces steroidal activity.

Recent research has uncovered evidence of interactions between the steroid response element RXRs with another superfamily of protein-activated receptors—peroxisome-proliferated activated receptors (PPARs). PPARs are currently of special interest as a potential cure for diabetes, reducing blood lipids and cholesterol, as well as losing body fat.

When activated, certain PPAR groups such as PPAR alpha or PPAR gamma can help increase insulin sensitivity and alter the composition of adipose fat tissue, respectively. The interaction of PPARs with steroidal receptor elements to form heterodimers, which affect insulin receptors and fat tissue composition, leads to the conclusion that steroid hormone interactions go far beyond their traditional perceived functions as growth, sex, and stress regulators. The steroid hormone receptor-related nucleotic activity interacts with other hormones' nucleic sites to induce a powerful biological impact on fat-burning, anti-aging, and protection from metabolic decline.

Steroid Hormones: Practical Notes

- Undereating and exercising stimulate steroid hormone synthesis in steroid hormone-producing cells (via cellular factor cAMP).
- Maintaining optimum cholesterol levels helps optimize steroid hormone production.
- Liver detoxification, avoidance of estrogenic chemicals, fat loss, and maintaining normal levels of androgens (avoiding chronic overspiking of androgen level via supplements or drugs) all help prevent over-expression of the aromatase enzyme complex (conversion of testosterone to estrogen).
- Eating high-potassium food activates aldosterone, with its probable survival-related primal muscle-toning potential.
- High energy turnover: Periodic cycles of exercise and undereating followed by relaxation and overeating will help enhance the overall metabolic rate while increasing steroid hormone activity.
- Incorporating intense pre-workout shock sets followed by intense and long supersets, along with forced sets in workout routines with short rest intervals between sets, can help take advantage of the cortisol wave, thereby establishing better anabolic potential during exercise as well as improving resistance to stress.
- Complete nutrition and sufficient calories are critically important for proper steroidal activity.
- Chronic calorie restrictions and low-fat and low-carb diets may suppress steroid production and thereby adversely affect libido, physical performance, and overall conditioning.

The next chapter, Chapter 4, covers the anabolic actions of dietary fatty acids and the crucial role they play in regulating steroidogenesis (steroid hormone synthesis). The chapter also offers practical advice about how to take advantage of dietary fats for promoting muscular development.

Dietary Fats for Repair and Growth

F atty acids have a profound effect on muscle gain and fat loss. Fat is the building block of all cell membranes. It is the precursor for all steroid hormones and some neurotransmitters. Unknown to many people, fat is also a preferred fuel for skeletal muscles. Most importantly, certain fatty acids can generate a hormone-like effect on the body, regulating anabolic and catabolic actions.

This chapter covers the anabolic actions of essential fatty acids (EFAs). Whether one gains or wastes muscle depends on the pro-inflammatory and anti-inflammatory actions of EFAs. Dietary fat composition can affect the direction of many metabolic actions, including muscle gain and fat loss. Although fatty acids have earned a reputation as being either good or bad, those judgments are sometimes misleading, particularly with regard to muscle gain and fat loss. The question of what is "good" and what is "bad" needs to be readdressed.

Good Fats, Bad Fats

Every drama plays the good guys against the bad guys. We see the drama play out in politics, in history, and in our everyday lives. Our ideas about what is good or bad change according to the times in which we live and the individual circumstances of our lives. What is considered good now may be considered bad later, and vice versa.

The notion that there are good fats that can heal and bad fats that can kill fires the imagination: We thrill to the idea of a dramatic struggle between the forces of good and evil. Who will be the ultimate victor? Because of our uncertainty and fear of death from what we perceive as "bad fats," many of us have developed obsessive fat phobias and thus attempt to avoid eating fat-rich foods. Among health-conscious consumers, meat and whole-dairy consumption has declined significantly, and sales of low-fat foods have reached record highs.

Beliefs about the biological actions of fatty acids as being good or bad seem to have originated from a disease perspective. Since heart and blood pressure diseases are always associated with inflammation and pain, any anti-inflammatory substance whether synthetic or natural has been considered to be solely beneficial, whereas any pro-inflammatory agent has been considered harmful and bad. However, life is not a disease and human beings need not approach their daily diets as a crisis management. The fact that something is considered beneficial to a sick body does not mean that it is necessarily good for a healthy body, and vice versa.

Food for Sex and Muscles

Although nowadays meat and cheese are often regarded as fattening and harmful foods, these same foods were once regarded as the great strength builders. Note that unlike other predators, humans are not inherently efficient in utilizing meat. Humans and all other primates are lacking certain enzymes that convert degraded proteins (D proteins) back to live and viable proteins (L proteins). Other animals such as canines and felines do have these "predator enzymes" and are better adapted to eating meat than humans. Nevertheless, historically meat has been regarded as most precious food. Ancient Greeks and Spartans considered meat to be the food for warriors.

Anthropologists have suggested that the human body hasn't changed much since the Stone Age. There is evidence that modern humans are still biologically designed to benefit from a hunter-gatherer diet naturally rich in high-fat foods.

Nuts, seeds, meat, eggs, and dairy have traditionally been regarded as vigor- and potency-enhancing foods. On the other hand, the meat-less, dairyless vegan diet has earned the reputation of being a healthy diet but not a "sexy"diet. The truth is that there are distinct dietary factors that affect sexuality regardless of whether or one is a meat-eater or a vegan.

Nuts, seeds, meat, eggs, and dairy foods do contain something that affects vigor and potency. This certain something also plays a critical role in numerous biological functions, including muscle gain and fat loss. This something is called functional fat.

In the body, fat plays a complex role that involves the ability to generate energy, cope with stress, and better survive. The ability to endure stress and hardship has kept humans alive during difficult conditions that involve physical threats, danger, and famine. This survival mechanism is partially regulated by the actions of certain oil components called essential fatty acids (EFAs). Essential fatty acids are the most functional fats in the body, regulating numerous metabolic actions that keep us alive. The word "essential" here means that EFAs cannot be produced by the body and therefore must be ingested from a dietary source.

To deliver their actions, EFAs must first convert into their active, hormone-like derivatives called prostaglandins (PGs). EFAs produce both pro-inflammatory and anti-inflammatory prostaglandins. Prostaglandins are divided into three major groups: PG Series 1 and 3 prostaglandins, which are mostly anti-inflammatory and therefore considered "good"; and PG Series 2 prostaglandins, which are mostly pro-inflammatory and therefore considered "bad."

Ironically, it is the allegedly bad prostaglandins that are immediately involved in our first reactions to stress. The pro-inflammatory prostaglandins help protect the body from physical stress and potential injury by activating a swift immune response and establishing an instant growth stimulation for tissue repair and recuperation.

The essential fatty acid that triggers pro-inflammatory growth-stimulating actions is called arachidonic acid (AA), the product of an omega-6 fat found abundantly in meat, egg yolk, and dairy. AA is considered the "worst" of all the bad guys. Nutrition experts warn of AA's dangerous effects by linking it with cardiovascular disease and cancer. When overly expressed, AA may indeed increase the risk of cancer, but so do all of the most potent anabolic agents, including growth hormone growth factors and testosterone.

Arachidonic acid stimulates the production of steroid hormones through a special regulatory protein called steroidogenic acute regulatory protein (StAR). This protein plays a critical role in stimulating steroid biosynthesis. Its main action involves facilitating the transfer of cholesterol to the inner mitochondrial membrane in steroid hormone-producing cells, thus accelerating steroid hormone synthesis. AA stimulates growth in more than one way. More on this soon.

Anti- and Pro-Inflammatory Prostaglandins		
Anti-inflammatory	Series 1	DGLA-derived
Anti-inflammatory	Series 3	EPA DHA-derived
Inflammatory	Series 2	Arachidonic acid

Anti-Inflammatory Drugs and Painkillers Suppress Growth

We've learned that adrenal hormones play a critical role in regulating reactions to stress. Recent cancer research reveals the important regulatory role of beta adrenoreceptors in the activation and release of arachidonic acid. Experiments conducted in 2001 at the College of Veterinary Medicine at the University of Tennessee, Knoxville, revealed that adrenergic agonists caused the release of AA and stimulated DNA synthesis, while beta-blockers, COX inhibitors, or LOX inhibitors blocked this growth-stimulating effect.[3]

It is reasonable to assume that there is a strong survival mechanism involving pro-inflammatory growth-stimulating agents that can help the body recuperate from stress-related catabolic crises and get even tougher and stronger by building new tissue. This survival-related reaction to stress involves all anabolic agents, including steroids, prostaglandins, cytokines, adrenal hormones, cellular factor cAMP, and growth hormone. People who take anti-inflammatory drugs or painkillers should be aware that these drugs antagonize this survival mechanism by inhibiting pro-inflammatory prostaglandins and thus significantly suppress growth.

How do anti-inflammatory drugs inhibit growth?

Arachidonic acid arises from gamma linoleic acid, an essential omega-6 derivative. The AA is then metabolized to become part of the cell membrane lipids. AA is released from the cell membrane by the enzyme phospholipase A2. This enzyme is activated by a variety of external stimuli, such as during exercise via adrenaline, and is inhibited by corticosteroid hormones and anti-inflammatory drugs. This inhibitory effect of cortisol on AA release may partly explain why anti-inflammatory drugs and cortisol have a suppressive effect on muscle gain. The enzymes that synthesize prostaglandins from AA are called COX 1 and COX 2. Anti-inflammatory drugs such as aspirin and other nonsteroidal anti-inflammatory drugs (NSAIDs) are all COX inhibitors. Anti-inflammatory drugs, including over-the-counter NSAIDs, have been known to inhibit AA actions. Athletes and bodybuilders who take anti-inflammatory drugs and painkillers should be aware of the potential inhibitory effect of these drugs on muscular development.

Growth-Inhibiting EFAs

Both essential fatty acids—omega-3 and omega-6—are considered vital and beneficial. Nevertheless, omega-3 EFA is featured as the current favorite in diet books. Fish oil rich in the omega-3 fatty acids EPA and DHA is one of the most popular nutritional products sold in health food stores and pharmacies.

Omega-3 EFA is actively involved in critical biological functions such as improving cognitive abilities, alleviating pain and inflammation, lowering blood pressure and cholesterol, improving insulin sensitivity, and inhibiting over-estrogenic activity, thus suppressing tumor formation.

However, as beneficial as omega-3 EFAs are, one may wonder if they are always as good as they seem.

By the 1930s, scientists had discovered that certain prostaglandins that reduce pain and inflammation also inhibit the mobilization of fatty acids from adipose tissue for energy. In other words, when imbalanced, certain anti-inflammatory prostaglandins that are considered "good" may suppress the body's ability to burn fat. Obviously, this is not good news for people who want to lean down.

Additionally, omega-3 fatty acids may inhibit adrenal actions. Adrenal hormones activate cellular factor cAMP, which is necessary for all cellular anabolic-stimulating actions and fat-burning. Moreover, both adrenal hormones and arachidonic acid are somehow involved in the stimulation of steroid hormone actions necessary for muscular recuperation and development. That adrenal arachidonic acid-related process may be interrupted by the actions of omega-3 EFAs. It is now known that omega-3 fatty acids work as beta-blockers, blocking the beta-adrenoreceptors similar to the way beta-blocker drugs work. Omega-3 EFAs can help lower cardiac stress and reduce blood pressure; however, their medicinal effect may ironically antagonize growth and fat-burning. Note that all beta-blocker drugs cause side effects, including decreased libido and impaired sexual performance.

EFA Balance: The Most Critical Contributing Factor for Maximum Performance

Omega-3 and omega-6 EFAs balance each other's actions. In fact, pro- and anti-inflammatory prostaglandins help maintain healthy metabolic processes that involve an immediate inflammatory response to stress, such as during exercise, followed by an anti-inflammatory secondary response that reduces inflammation and facilitates final recuperation processes that include tissue repair and muscle development. As you can see, both omega-6 and omega-3 fatty acids are critically important.

Both inflammatory and anti-inflammatory prostaglandins are inherently beneficial, and both are necessary for optimal health. As previously stated, the alleged bad guys help stimulate growth potential, whereas the alleged good guys help facilitate the initial growth potential that leads to actual tissue recuperation, repair, and development.

Once in balance, dietary EFAs are likely to grant a healthy and vibrant metabolism. However, an imbalance or deficiency of EFAs can lead to chronic over-expression of one EFA over another. Dietary EFA imbalance can cause chronic over-activity of either pro- or anti-inflammatory prostaglandins, an adverse and potentially destructive condition that may lead to chronic disease or an overall metabolic breakdown. Note that in spite of the current hype on fish oils, omega-3 deficiencies are still common in our society. The excess of omega-6 oils in our diet (via vegetable oils such as corn, canola, safflower, and soy) often cause an imbalance of omega-6 over omega-3 EFAs in the body. An excess of omega-6 is known for promoting excess of estrogen, metabolic disorders, and cancer in animals and humans.

EFA Ratios for Reducing Inflammation, Sensitizing Insulin, and Gaining Muscle

Maintaining a proper balance between dietary omega-6 and omega-3 EFAs is of the utmost importance in reducing inflammation, sensitizing insulin, and sustaining peak physical conditioning.

Essential fatty acids are the building blocks of cell membranes. The cell membrane is a barrier characterized by highly selective permeability. It is involved in the process of energy transformation and cellular communication through special membrane receptors that are sensitive to external stimuli. The cell membrane consists of a double layer of phospholipids containing both omega-6 and omega-3 fatty acids, including AA, DHA, and EPA. These long-chain polyunsaturated fatty acids contribute to the flexibility and viability of the cell's membrane. Flexibility of cell membranes is critical for proper receptor binding, ionic flow, and overall regulation of energy production and growth. EFA deficiencies or EFA imbalance can lead to impaired cellular metabolism that may adversely manifest as insulin insensitivity, impaired energy utilization, fat gain, and cessation of growth.

As a rule, people who suffer from acute or chronic inflammation resulting from disease, injury, or post-exercise reaction should increase their consumption of omega-3 oil. Omega-3 EFAs are found abundantly in flaxseed oil, hemp oil, and fish oil. The same advice applies to people who suffer from insulin resistance. Omega-3 oil has been shown to help improve insulin sensitivity. Individuals who suffer from inflammation or insulin resistance may benefit from keeping a high dietary ratio of omega-3 to omega-6 fatty acid (2:1 or 3:1).

People interested in maximizing growth should employ a ratio that is somewhat higher in omega-6 fatty acid than in omega-3 fatty acid by simply adding more AA-rich foods such as eggs and dairy as sources for protein and fat. For muscle gain, good old-fashioned dairy and eggs are still the choice of warriors! Regardless of what you might have heard about the dangers of eating whole dairy and eggs (with the yolk), with their high cholesterol and saturated fats, these foods were and still are the most viable choices for overall potency and muscle power. The so-called bad fat in animal food is partially responsible for its potent anabolic properties. Foods rich in arachidonic acid such as eggs and dairy products should therefore be considered most beneficial for the purpose of muscle gain. Other fat-rich foods that promote sexuality and muscularity are raw nuts and seeds. Besides their high mineral, amino acid, vitamin, and antioxidant content, they are rich in certain fatty compounds called phytosterols that have been shown to lower cholesterol and promote production of steroid hormones.

If you are a "meat-and-potatoes" type, you should take advantage of the pro-anabolic high ratio of AA consumption. However, to prevent the over-expression of AA-derived prostaglandins that may lead to chronic inflammation and result in overall metabolic decline and muscle waste, be sure to balance your diet with foods rich in omega-3, such as fish, seafood, flaxseed, or hempseed or their derived oils. Always bear in mind that animal-derived foods (other than seafood) are very low in omega-3 EFAs and that supplementing animal-based diets with omega-3 oils is highly recommended. Above all else, be sure to apply this information according to your specific needs.

"Bad Fat" Can Help Build Muscle

This section details the anabolic actions of arachidonic acid (AA) and may be of particular interest to athletes and bodybuilders. The practical advice may help maximize the anabolic effects of exercise. AA is the dominant prostaglandin precursor. AA-derived prostaglandins are generally more active than prostaglandins derived from other essential fatty acids (EFAs). AA-derived prostaglandins generate their complex actions on numerous cellular processes that activate special growth-mediating proteins, including heat-shock proteins, mitogen-activated protein kinases, and enzymes that eventually stimulate anabolic steroid hormones and growth actions on exercising muscles.

This complex of actions, mediated by AA, helps maintain muscle protein integrity during exposure to exercise-related stress and heat, and facilitates anabolic actions that help improve muscle composition and increase muscle mass.

Stress stimuli, such as that induced during exercise or a physical injury, increases arachidonic acid release from the cell membrane through phosphorylation of the cytosolic enzyme phospholipase A2. This enzymatic activation is induced by stress-activated protein kinases (SAPKs), which themselves are activated during inflammatory processes, typically during exercise, by cytokines (which are AA derivatives), phospholipids, polysaccharides, and stress stimuli such as heat and free radicals (mostly considered "bad guys"). Generally, SAPK is a growth inhibitor that is likely to balance other stress-related growth-stimulating agents. However, SAPK 2 helps induce phosphorylation and activation of heat-shock protein 27, a fact that may play an important role in the mechanism that repairs damaged muscle tissues and thereby helps cell survival and muscular maintenance under stress.

The conversion of arachidonic acid into its active prostaglandins occurs in a certain chamber of the cell membrane (called the endoplasmic reticulum) by a complex of enzymes that include COX 1 and COX 2. Arachidonic acid plays a critical role in survival under stress or physical trauma. Under normal circumstances, AA-related inflammatory response has a protective and beneficial function.

The release of AA increases the actions of inflammatory mediators such as cytokines, interleukins, and tumor necrosis factor, which have a strong immuno-boosting impact on the body and help suppress bacterial or viral infections while enhancing overall detection of sick and damaged cells.

Italian researchers have indeed found that during inflammation, activated macrophages secrete certain growth factors similar to the cytokines that promote muscle growth.[4] However, the inflammatory process can be a double-edged sword when the inflammatory response becomes chronic or exaggerated, it leads to inflammatory diseases such as rheumatoid arthritis, Crohn's disease, or heart disease. If untreated, chronic inflammation can also lead to waste of muscle tissues. Thus arachidonic acid can either save you or waste you.

Inflammation is a natural defense reaction to physical stress or injury. Inflammatory reactions are often associated with catabolic processes that involve wasting of tissues such as muscles and bones. Oftentimes, during stress-related catabolic tissue degradation, the body attempts to compensate by activating the most powerful growth-stimulating agents such as cellular factor cyclic AMP (cAMP) and the release of arachidonic acid with its related active pro-anabolic prostaglandins and cytokines.

That is what happens during intense exercise: Intense resistance or explosive and speed-related training are in fact catabolic activities that initially tear muscle fiber and connective tissue. The activation of pro-inflammatory prostaglandins and cytokines combined with adrenaline and its related energizing impact gives the body the necessary arsenal to compensate and build stronger muscle and bones, thus preparing the body to handle further stress more efficiently.

Practical Conclusions

In practical terms, one can facilitate AA actions simply by consuming foods rich in AA such as meat, eggs, and dairy products. However, the conversion of omega-6 oils (linoleic acid) into their more active gamma linoleic acid form, from which arachidonic acid is derived, is often inhibited as a result of various metabolic factors, including high blood sugar, zinc deficiencies, vitamin deficiencies, and aging. Supplementing one's intake with dietary sources rich in gamma linoleic acid, such as primrose oil or black currant oil, can help to bypass this weak enzymatic process.

AA biosynthesis can also be suppressed through the use of oils rich in omega-3 EFA, including flaxseed, hempseed, and fish oils. Thus, to establish anabolic potential, it is important to maintain a balance between omega-6 and omega-3 EFAs.

Most people are deficient in omega-3 oils. Therefore, the high ratio of omega-6 to omega-3 may cause imbalance and metabolic disorders among "meat and potatoes" guys. Beef-eaters may need to supplement their diet with omega-3 oils to protect against AA over-expression that can lead to chronic inflammation and may result in disease and muscle wasting.

CHAPTER 5

Growth Hormone

Known as "the hormone of youth," with its reputation of being a tissue builder and a fat burner, growth hormone (GH) is the subject of much scientific research today, though it remains a mystery to most people. The purpose of this chapter is to present the true facts behind growth hormone and provide practical guidelines to individuals who are interested in naturally taking advantage of this hormone to get leaner, stronger, and healthier.

In order to effectively boost growth hormone, one needs to learn when and how it is secreted and what really triggers its levels to rise. The secretion of GH is controlled by many variables including food intake, exercise, sleep, stress, age, body mass, and gender. Most importantly, the secretion of growth hormone is profoundly affected by the circadian clock. As you'll soon learn, GH is mostly a nocturnal (nightly) hormone, but other factors including hunger, physical stress, and power naps can up-regulate the release of GH.

Blood levels of GH are characterized by large pulses followed by very low pulses. The largest pulse occurs during deep sleep at night. GH secretion may be adversely affected by poor eating habits, sleep deprivation, chronic stress, low thyroid activity, and certain drugs. A GH deficiency can lead to abnormal body fat, a decrease in exercise endurance, poor health, reduced bone mineral density, impaired lipid metabolism, stunted growth, and accelerated aging. Proper manipulation of feeding and sleeping cycles has been shown to significantly enhance the actions of GH.

Growth Hormone Basics

Growth hormone reaches its peak level during deep sleep. To understand how sleep induces maximum GH impact, it is essential to understand the basics of the sleep-wake cycle.

The sleep cycle consists of two distinct sleep stages: rapid eye movement (REM) sleep and non-REM sleep. Non-REM sleep can be further divided into light and deep sleep. Deep, non-REM sleep can be discerned by a high-amplitude low-frequency delta wave. This is why deep, non-REM sleep is called slow-wave sleep.

The sleep-wake cycle is divided into three stages: non-REM sleep, REM sleep, and wakefulness. Sleep is generally evaluated according to two criteria: (first) timing and (second) duration. Sleep is controlled by neuropeptides and hormones that are secreted by the hypothalamus-pituitary-adrenal axis. In fact, neuropeptides and hormones that regulate sleep, wakefulness, feeding, and stress also play important roles in a feedback control that regulates GH secretion through stimulation and inhibition.

Growth hormone-releasing hormone (GHRH) and deep sleep promote one another. High levels of GHRH can increase the length of deep sleep, and low levels can impair slow-wave sleep, thus shortening sleep time. Interestingly, the amount of GHRH mRNA could be highest in the morning, particularly for people who suffer from insomnia or those who retire late. Thus, for some individuals, skipping morning sleep impairs GH secretion. For both of these groups, an afternoon nap is highly recommended. The body compensates for lack of deep sleep by inducing it more efficiently during the afternoon siesta.

Growth hormone, also called somatotropin, is a polypeptide hormone consisting of 191 amino acids in humans. GH-secreting cells called somatotropic cells are found in the anterior pituitary. The main effects of GH are stimulation of bone growth, anabolic effect in the muscles, conservation of protein and carbohydrates, and mobilization of fat for energy (lipolysis).

The effects of GH are partially mediated by metabolic "agents" called somatomedins, of which the most important are the insulin-like growth factors IGF1 and IGF2. Plasma (circulating) IGFs primarily originate in the liver and kidneys; however, IGF somatomedins are produced locally by several other tissues including the muscle. As noted, secretion of GH from the anterior pituitary is pulsatile: The secretion bursts are followed by nearly undetectable levels of plasma GH.

Females have higher plasma levels of GH than do males, who have fewer GH pulses, but male GH pulses are of higher amplitude. Growth hormone secretion is controlled by an inner circadian rhythm and starts to decline during the fourth decade of life. It is important to note that aging diminishes GH secretion during the daily hours first, while the nightly sleep-associated GH pulse persists longer. Thus, any method that can help increase GH release during the day will most likely have a profound anti-aging effect. What is the trick? The answer is astonishingly simple, and it doesn't require spending money on GH-boosting supplements or taking drugs.

Keep reading and you'll understand how certain manipulations of meal timing, hunger, exercise, and sleep are key influencing factors in maximizing GH impact on the body. The upcoming pages reveal how to take advantage of GH to turn on a most powerful survival switch that accelerates fat-burning and the presence of spare protein in the muscle. Let's see how GH works.

GH and Dopamine for Sustaining Potency and Muscularity

Growth hormone works in sync with the brain neurohormone dopamine to sustain cognitive functions, energy, and virility in men and women. GHRH (growth hormone-releasing hormone) stimulates GH secretion, but most importantly it is also involved in other critical actions that help sustain the body's virility and vitality. Apparently GHRH and dopamine couple to protect virility and to maintain muscularity. GHRH cells produce dopamine as a co-neurotransmitter. This is critically important since dopamine inhibits thyroid-stimulating hormone (TSH) and prolactin, thus protecting the body from over-expression of the female lactating hormone. Prolactin is known for its antagonizing effect on male sex hormones and for causing feminization of the male body. High prolactin and TSH are anti-anabolic. Therefore GHRH, dopamine, and GH play critical roles in sustaining potency, virility, male physical characteristics, and overall muscularity. This same GH-dopamine impact can benefit the female body in a similar way: preventing excess of prolactin and thus sustaining optimum hormone balance and a healthy metabolism.

Stimulation and Inhibition of Growth Hormone

The release of GH is regulated by stimulating and inhibitory agents. Growth hormone-releasing hormone (GHRH), which stimulates GH secretion, is a peptide-stimulating hormone. It is stimulated by cellular factor cAMP, and its secretion increases when GH levels drop.

Somatostatin (somatotropin release-inhibiting factor) is a hormone-like peptide that inhibits GH secretion. Somatostatin is widely distributed in the body. The local release of somatostatin may protect the body from over-expression of GH, which could lead to growth of internal organs and cancer.

Growth hormone regulates its own blood level through a negative-feedback mechanism. Plasma levels of GH regulate the activity of somatostatin and GHRH cells. An elevated level of GH increases somatostatin release and decreases GHRH release. Conversely, a low level of GH decreases somatostatin and increases GHRH levels. As noted, GH levels are mediated indirectly by insulin-like growth factor (IGFs), neuropeptides, and adrenal and steroid hormones. Nevertheless, this autonegative feedback control of the GH-GHRH-somatostatin axis generates a rhythmic alternation between high and low GH levels.

GH Secretagogues

GH secretagogues (GHS) are a class of proteins and non-protein compounds known to be potent stimulators of GH release. Generally, GHS are also sleep inducers. In young adults, IGF1 levels increase as a result of GHS administration, and this increase relates to GHS' promoting effect on GH. There is great interest currently in synthetic GHS as a possible remedy for age-related GH deficiency. It is commonly believed that certain amino acids such as arginine, ornithine, and tryptophan may help increase GH release. However, no conclusive evidence exists that supplementation of free-form amino acids at bedtime helps increase GH activity. The effectiveness of commercial GH secretagogue products is often in serious doubt. Some products, however, have shown genuine stimulating effects on GH release during slow-wave sleep, but unfortunately, because of the possibility of misuse by some segments of the population (such as with rape drugs), these products are illegal in most states. Nonetheless, GH release is effectively stimulated by indigenous peptides that are produced in the body to regulate feeding cycles and hunger sensation. Galanin and neuropeptide Y are likely the most notable stimulators of GH release. Both neuropeptides that originally regulate feeding cycles can indirectly assist in muscle and strength gain. Other GH secretagogues are the peptides ghrelin and leptin, both of which relate to feeding cycles of dietary fat. Evidently there is a direct correlation between feeding and GH release. Let's see how all this really works.

Feeding Cycles and Growth Hormone

Food intake is an important influencing factor in growth rate. Mammalian feedings are controlled by an innate biological mechanism that regulates the species' capacity to initiate and stop feeding. Animals and humans eat to satisfy their immediate energy and nutritional needs. Regulation of food intake involves the sensation of external environmental factors such as food availability, danger, and even temperature. Under certain conditions such as lack of food or the presence of danger, human survival depends on the ability to endure nutritional stress by sustaining life through minimal food intake. Following a period of undereating, the body induces hunger along with the desire to overeat. Overeating allows the body to replenish and store energy and nutrients in anticipation of an upcoming high energy demand.

Animal and human feeding cycles are therefore primarily controlled by a survival mechanism that is triggered during conditions that involve fasting, undereating, or intense physical stress. Unknown to many, this survival mechanism stimulates powerful anabolic potential for compensation and adaptation. As you'll soon see, this awesome mechanism is surprisingly regulated via neuropeptides that signal hunger and satiety.

The brain plays a key role in regulating feeding cycles as well as rejuvenation of tissues and growth. Studies conducted in the 1940s showed that certain lesions in the hypothalamus reduce feeding, whereas other lesions induce overeating. Those findings led researchers to the hypothesis that humans are inherently programmed for feeding cycles based on periodic undereating and overeating. Recent biological techniques reveal a more sophisticated neural control of feeding and energy balance. There is growing evidence that a large number of neuropeptides exert either stimulatory or inhibitory effects on feeding, indirectly affecting growth and overall energy expenditure. Interestingly, some of these neuropeptides were found to exert their actions via stimulation of GH secretion. Let's examine how they work.

Neuropeptide Y and Galanin

Human feeding is controlled by hypothalamic neurons. The hypothalamic feeding control center receives stimulatory or inhibitory signals by neuropeptides and hormones. As previously mentioned, these signals are part of a survival mechanism that interacts with external environmental conditions. For instance, a lack of food increases hunger, stimulating peptides such as neuropeptide Y, galanin, and the stress hormone cortisol.

Conversely, when a full meal is consumed, hunger-inhibiting agents such as leptin and insulin normally signal the brain to sense satiety and reduce feeding. As you'll learn later on, this feeding mechanism is more than often interrupted by poor eating habits, with often severe and even mortal consequences. Most modern diets that incorporate frequent meals during the day disturb the body's ability to efficiently control healthy feeding cycles through primal sensations of hunger and satiety. When eating under constant stress such as during the active hours of the day, the body is overwhelmed by the adverse effects of the stress hormone cortisol.

Cortisol, a hunger-stimulating agent, opposes the inhibitory signals in the brain, thereby causing chronic cravings for food that often lead to compulsive bingeing and weight gain. Cycling between periods of undereating during the day and overeating at night will most likely help minimize stress-related cortisol impact when eating. Exercise can further benefit the body's ability to resist stress and regulate cortisol.

The survival-related feeding mechanism controls various biological functions. In addition to stimulating or inhibiting the amount of food eaten, neuropeptides help regulate eating behavior. Neuropeptide Y induces a preference for carbohydrates, whereas galanin induces a preference for fat. Neuropeptides that regulate feeding may also exert signals that promote anabolism or catabolism. Neuropeptide Y and galanin induce a general anabolic state by stimulating GH release, thus improving energy balance and accelerating lipolysis (fat-burning). Conversely, a chronic high plasma level of cortisol may adversely affect growth while increasing lipogenesis (fat gain).

Hunger and Growth

Most people today suffer from "hunger phobia." The fear of hunger makes people eat whatever and whenever. The current epidemic of obesity and other modern diseases may be related to the inability of modern people to take advantage of hunger. The following paragraphs will show you how hunger works in more than one way to benefit your life. Besides giving you the desire to eat, it also enhances your ability to get leaner, stronger, and healthier. Again, the following information may be a bit technical, but nevertheless it's important to clear this controversial topic.

Neuropeptide Y is found in the central nervous system and the gastrointestinal tract. In addition to its effect on feeding and energy balance, neuropeptide Y has been implicated in the regulation of circadian rhythms, reproduction, growth hormone secretion, cardiovascular function, anxiety, and memory.

Galanin is a peptide present in the gastrointestinal tract and widely in the central nervous system, where it participates in numerous brain functions such as feeding, memory, and hormone release. Both neuropeptide Y and galanin are believed to increase GH secretion by inhibiting the GH inhibitor somatostatin; neuropeptide Y and galanin promote GH secretion in other ways as well. They both inhibit noradrenergic cells in the locus coeruleus noradren region of the brain, thus further accelerating the inhibitory effect on somatostatin. (Noradrenergic cells promote somatostatin release, thus inhibiting GH secretion during the day.)

In summary, the hunger-neuropeptide-growth hormone axis may play a significant role in regulating feeding as well as growth. All the above information clearly indicates that hunger sensation, with its related neuropeptides, helps increase GH release during the day. The low levels of GH typically during the daily hours may have to do with the "lack of hunger" in our affluent society. As noted, human feeding cycles are controlled by a primal survival mechanism that helps sustain life under extreme conditions that involve lack of food or intense physical stress with high energy demand. Therefore, undereating and hunger turn on a powerful survival-related anabolic switch (via growth hormone release) that accelerates fat burning while sparing protein in the muscle.

Eating at night while relaxing finalizes the daily feeding cycle. Keeping a steady, daily sleep-wake cycle and avoiding sleep deprivation helps maximize the impact of GH on the body during deep sleep. Overall, maintaining feeding cycles that involve periods of hunger and physical stress (exercise) followed by periods of nourishment, satiety, and relaxation will grant healthy sleeping cycles while maximizing the anabolic and rejuvenating actions of growth hormone on the body.

Growth hormone has a profound affinity for bone and connective tissue buildup. Strength and high-impact athletes including powerlifters, martial artists, and football players often suffer from injuries resulting from weak tendons or low bone density. Bones and connective tissue play a critical role in muscular development. Growth hormone helps facilitate the repair of muscle fibers and tendons and the mineralization of bones. Insufficient growth hormone release impairs overall muscle and strength gain. Such deficiency also compromises the body's ability to burn fat, recuperate from physical stress, and resist aging.

CHAPTER 6

Insulin-Like Growth Factor 1

Insulin-like growth factors (IGFs) are known as growth-promoting mediators of growth hormone. Among them IGF1 is the most notable and potent growth factor. Insulin-like growth factor 1 (IGF1) is regarded as a powerful growth-inducing agent that has the fastest and most immediate anabolic impact on muscle tissue. IGF1 is a single-chain polypeptide. Like its name, IGF1 has insulin-like and growth factor-like effects on the muscle.

The IGF1 receptor (IGF-1R) is designed similar to the insulin receptor. Both have almost the same cell surface receptor with tyrosine kinase-related activities. The tyrosine kinase domains of IGF1 and insulin receptors possess similar structure and actions. Nonetheless, despite the high degree of homology, experimental evidence suggests that the two receptors have distinct biological roles. The insulin receptor is known to be a key regulator of glucose transport and biosynthesis of glycogen and fat, whereas the IGF1 receptor is a potent regulator of cell growth and differentiation. Note that similar to IGF1, insulin has an anabolic effect on muscle cells. Under specific metabolic conditions involving certain feeding cycles and a state of high insulin sensitivity, insulin can induce a potent growth factor-like impact. However, unlike IGF1, insulin's anabolic activities may involve undesirable fat gain.

IGF1 and Muscular Development

Insulin-like growth factors stimulate skeletal muscle growth and differentiation through a chain of cellular events. IGF's receptor is a transmembrane tyrosine kinase widely expressed in muscle tissue as well as other tissue and cell types. (This is a protein receptor on the cell's surface that works like a revolving door, allowing certain substances to penetrate the cell, interact, and induce their actions.) Activation of the receptor results from the binding of growth factor ligands IGF1 and IGF2. (IGF2 has a lower affinity than IGF1 and is therefore considered less potent.) IGF1's anabolic effect involves interactions with certain stress-activated proteins such as heat-shock proteins or stress-activated protein kinases. These proteins help regulate muscle reaction to physical stress by facilitating actions that promote maintenance, repair, growth, and differentiation. IGF1 also plays an important role in enhancing the expression of contractible proteins such as actin and myosin, thus helping increase muscle strength.

The binding of IGF1 to its receptor stimulates a cascade of phosphorylation events that interact with cellular proteins such as phosphatidyl inositol-3 kinase. It is the activation of the latter that leads to the ergogenic and anabolic effects of IGF1 such as enhanced glucose transport, enhanced myocyte contractibility, and inhibition of protein breakdown as well as inhibition of programmed cell death (apoptosis).

IGF1 and Muscular Differentiation

The process of muscular differentiation involves a molecular mechanism that switches the anabolic program from proliferation (increasing the number of cells) to differentiation (the fusion of precursor cells to muscle cells). Intensive studies have led to the discovery of transcriptional agents that play a pivotal role during differentiation. One of these muscle growth and differentiation agents consists of a family of proteins called myogenic regulatory factors (MRFs)—in particular, the protein myogenin, expressed exclusively in skeletal muscles. IGF1 stimulates muscle differentiation and growth by the induction of myogenin mRNA (activating the genes that produce myogenin) as well as other growth-promoting protein kinases via activation of the previously mentioned phosphatidyl inositol-3 kinase. IGF's growth-stimulating impact manifests through different intracellular signaling pathways. One of them is the mitogen-activated protein kinase. As noted previously, mitogen-activated protein kinase is activated during exercise via pro-inflammatory prostaglandins. The activation of this protein may be responsible for the growth impact of IGF1 during and after intense physical exercise.

IGF1 and Heat-Shock Proteins

As noted, IGF1 up-regulates the actions of the stress proteins, heat-shock protein 27 (HSP-27), and stress-activated protein kinase 2 (SAPK2). Heat-shock proteins have been some of the most well-preserved proteins throughout evolution. Under severe physiological stress, these proteins fulfill essential functions in cells, protecting them from irreversible damage. HSP-27 has been found to be involved in thermotolerance, differentiation, and proliferation of muscle cells. Most importantly, HSP-27 helps protect muscle structural integrity, thus improving muscle response to stress and accelerating recuperation.

Overall, IGF1 induces a potent anabolic state in muscles, especially during intense physical stress. Interacting with stress-activated proteins, pro-inflammatory prostaglandins, cytokines, and other stress-related growth promoters such as nitric oxide and cellular factor cAMP, IGF1 is likely the fastest and most compelling growth factor that effectively helps protect muscles from stress-related damage while stimulating growth, differentiation, and increased strength.

All the information above applies to normal conditions, under which IGF1 and its mediators help protect the body (in particular the muscles) from damage, enhancing adaptation of muscles to stress via growth and strengthening. However, over-expression of IGFs and stress-activated protein may lead to uncontrolled proliferation of cells and cancer.

As potent as it is, intravenous injections of IGF1 can be fatal. On the other hand, natural methods that enhance the actions of growth hormone and IGFs could be most effective in establishing a potent anabolic state, supporting the immune system and helping slow the aging process.

Natural Methods to Enhance IGF1 Actions

- Periodic fasting, undereating, and exercise may help stimulate IGF1 and increase its receptors in muscles.
- Post-exercise carbohydrate consumption is recommended for maximizing IGF1 anabolic actions (via insulin interference).
- Complete nutritional meals and a sufficient calorie intake are necessary for overall growth.
- Minimizing carb consumption to one meal per day, or right after exercise, as well as increasing consumption of omega-3 essential fatty acids, may benefit in two ways: first, protect against insulin resistance and second, enhance anabolic actions (more on the correlation between IGF1 and insulin later—see Chapter 10).

CHAPTER 7

The Anabolic Cycle: Timing Is Everything

Professional athletes, powerlifters, bodybuilders, and veteran martial artists know that real gains in muscle and strength require time. While fat-burning is a process that can be initiated instantly through diet and exercise, muscular growth is a slower event that takes place in an interval-like manner. Understanding this is crucial for effective muscular development.

An anabolic event occurs in two stages. The first stage is growth stimulation, and the second is growth finalization. The growth stimulation stage involves the actions of hormones and compounds that stimulate growth, including the peptide-stimulating hormones (LH and GHRH), adrenal hormones, cellular factor cAMP, and prostaglandins.

The second stage, growth finalization, is the materializing stage that facilitates actual muscle gain. This stage involves the actions of steroids and growth hormone that were previously stimulated by the first stage of the anabolic cycle. The amount of time it takes to complete both stages of the anabolic cycle is the amount of time required for effective muscular development.

Muscle gain occurs under the following three conditions:

1. Hormones: induction of the "hormone cocktail" that includes steroids, GH, IGF1, thyroid, and insulin.
2. Nutrition: complete and sufficient nutrition that includes all essential proteins, fatty acids, vitamins, minerals, and antioxidants. Carbs should also be regarded as both anabolic and anti-catabolic food for muscles.

3. Energy: High cellular energy is required for the repair and buildup of muscle tissue.

If one of the above conditions is compromised—whether it's a hormonal deficiency, insufficient nutrition, or low cellular energy—growth will be severely impaired.

Muscular development is part of a survival mechanism that originally helped animals and humans adapt to physical stress and hardship. Each of us carries an inner code that governs our reactions to environmental changes. Most primitive, single-cell organisms such as amoebae or bacteria respond to changes in their external environment (for example, temperature or food availability). More advanced multicellular living organisms such as animals and humans must also respond to changes in their environment to stay alive.

Human survival depends on an elaborate network of cellular communication. Different signaling agents require different threshold times to induce their related actions. The duration varies over which signaling agent actions occur. Some actions, such as those of prostaglandins, take a fraction of a second, whereas others, such as steroid actions, last hours or even days. In other words, growth agents have either an immediate or a delayed impact on the body. Understanding this is critical for ultimately inducing muscle gain.

Short and Long Anabolic Impacts

The different time periods required for various hormones to induce their actions is the very factor that dictates the manner and duration of growth. Learning the time-impact factor can help you take advantage of the anabolic cycle to effectively induce muscular development.

As mentioned, hormones and their actions have a short or a long-lasting impact on the body. Certainly those hormones that have a short effect are often capable of generating an immediate impact on the body. On the other hand, hormones that have a long-lasting anabolic impact often deliver it in a delayed manner.

Swift impacts on the body are generated by peptide hormones including the adrenal hormones, insulin, and stimulating hormones such as ACTH, LH, and GHRH, whereas long-lasting but delayed impacts are generated by steroid hormones. The actions of cellular factor cAMP and prostaglandins depend on their related inducers, the adrenal hormones and EFA, respectively. For that matter, the impact of cAMP clearly depends on adrenal actions. Since adrenal actions are immediate and short, so are the effects of cAMP. However, certain conditions such as fasting and exercise substantially prolong adrenal actions and their related cAMP impact.

As for prostaglandins, even though their impact occurs in a split second, the accumulating effect of EFAs on prostaglandin production can facilitate a long-lasting effect.

To prevent any confusion, here is a brief summary:

Adrenal hormones, peptide-stimulating hormones, cAMP, and prostaglandins have an immediate and short impact that can last a split second to minutes to hours. Nonetheless, that impact can be prolonged under certain physiological conditions that involve fasting, undereating, and exercise. Steroid hormones have a delayed yet profound impact that can last for hours or even days.

Manipulating the Anabolic Cycle

The immediate but short-lived actions of stimulating hormones certainly indicate that the first stimulating stage of the anabolic cycle is fast but short and fragile. On the other hand, the delayed but long-lasting impact of steroid hormones indicates that while the second stage is slow, it can actually persist for days. Nonetheless, as you'll soon see, the long and profound anabolic actions of steroid hormones clearly depend on the preliminary short but fragile stimulating effect.

Often people fail to fully activate the first stage of the anabolic cycle. This preliminary stimulatory stage is quite unstable and can be abandoned as soon as it begins.

Physically active individuals who have poor eating habits and follow incorrect exercise routines, often lacking intensity and complexity, miss the opportunity to establish a viable growth stimuli. As a result, they are unable to reach the second conclusive stage of the anabolic cycle, and fail to gain the muscle and strength they desire.

The use of anabolic drugs is a way of bypassing the first stimulating stage of the anabolic cycle. However, every shortcut has its price. The dark side of anabolic drugs is well known and well documented. Aside from shattering the body's own production of hormones, anabolic drugs can adversely affect blood pressure, liver cholesterol, and lipid metabolism, and can cause over-expression of the aromatase enzyme with devastating estrogenic effects on the body. Other side effects include hair loss, acne, cancer, and growth of internal organs (such as abnormal growth of heart or intestines). Following the anabolic cycle naturally with no shortcuts is obviously a slower process but certainly much more effective in the long run.

Exercise and Rest

Chronic activation of hormones such as adrenals and stress-related hormones without proper rest may waste all available hormonal reserves and lead to adrenal exhaustion and hormonal insufficiency. Symptoms of such conditions include compromised reactions to stress, diminished thyroid functions, suppressed libido, and impaired growth.

Cycling between periods of action and rest is therefore necessary to effectively reach anabolic states. Length of training and exercise intensity are both important factors in inducing growth stimulation. In any case, rest and relaxation intervals are as important as workout sessions. Although exercise activates the first stage of the anabolic cycle, rest combined with proper nutrition closes the cycle and activates the second (final) stage, which facilitates the actual growth. As noted previously, one of the most important anabolic effects occurs at night during deep sleep, when growth hormone release reaches its peak level.

How to Take Advantage of the Anabolic Cycle

You can maximize the first stage of the anabolic cycle through under-eating and exercise. This combination will induce maximum growth stimulation via a complex of hormones, growth factors, and cellular factors. Adrenal hormone actions coupled with cAMP's stimulating effect on GH release and its related growth factors will help grant an immediate anabolic potential with a bonus of breaking fat storage for energy.

An excellent recommendation is to minimize carbohydrate consumption during the day. Doing so will prevent long-lasting insulin spikes during the daily hours that may suppress GH release and thus compromise the preliminary growth-stimulating process. Frequent carb feeding has been shown to cause insulin resistance (when insulin receptors become less effective in mobilizing glucose for energy), which is a major obstacle to muscle gain and fat loss. As you'll see soon, insulin plays an important role in the anabolic process by finalizing the actions of GH and IGF1 after exercise.

During the first stage of the anabolic cycle, insulin should be tightly controlled. Insulin antagonizes cAMP actions and is therefore likely to suppress its initial but critical growth-stimulating effect. However, since insulin has a profound anabolic effect during the second stage of the anabolic cycle, ingestion of carbs after exercise or during the evening meal can help finalize some critical anabolic actions that require insulin interference to be fully effective.

For muscle gain, it is vitally important to properly induce the first stimulating stage. Undereating combined with short, intense training sessions is probably the most efficient method of enforcing this short-lived, fragile stage of the anabolic cycle. Failing to establish a strong anabolic stimulating effect will undoubtedly reduce your opportunity to establish a potent anabolic state.

Incorporating recovery meals after exercise and overeating at night via big meals that include the correct EFA ratio, sufficient and complete protein supply, and enough calories to grant maximum cellular energy is likely to help facilitate the second anabolic state. Note that the above growth cycle can take a couple of days. This practical method of inducing the two critical stages of the anabolic cycle day in and day out (stimulating and finalizing anabolic states) is the only natural way to increase the probability of muscle and strength gain. However, like any other biological process, the anabolic cycle can potentially benefit from practical adjustments.

Simply stated, all of us, men and women alike, have our own genetic predispositions and unique needs. People have different metabolic demands and therefore require specific dietary and exercise modifications that will address their unique needs. Since we've already covered the role of EFAs in regulating growth, let me mention again that both omega-6 and omega-3 fatty acids are necessary for completion of the anabolic process; however, the ratio is adjusted according to a person's individual needs.

While arachidonic acid helps in signaling growth stimulation through pro-inflammatory prostaglandins and cytokines, during exercise omega-3 long-chain fatty acids DHA and EPA help stabilize insulin and reduce liver and blood cholesterol, thus improving fat utilization and steroid hormone synthesis. Most importantly, omega-3 oils and their active derivatives help balance the actions of AA, thus protecting the body from overmanifestation of AA that may lead to chronic inflammation and eventually to muscle waste.

People who use anabolic drugs may need to increase their consumption of omega-3 oil to help protect the body from fatty liver disease or cancer. Individuals who are insulin-resistant or diabetic could benefit from the same. However, over-consumption of omega-3 in relation to omega-6 (which rarely happens because most people suffer from omega-3 deficiencies) may adversely affect fat loss. In any case, it is important to maintain the correct ratio of omega-6 to omega-3, and to consume EFAs (particularly omega-3) in sufficient amounts. The body's requirements for omega-3 EFA dramatically increase on workout days. There is evidence that muscle omega-3 EFA content dramatically decreases in only one hour of intense drill. Omega-3 deficiencies are correlated with chronic inflammation and delayed muscle recuperation.

Eat to Gain

Bodybuilders and athletes should consider meat, dairy, and eggs to be the most anabolic foods. Nonetheless, since the biological value of meat protein is far inferior to dairy and eggs, it is recommended that the latter be primary sources of protein. Arachidonic acid, which is abundant in meat, dairy, and eggs, helps to induce initial anabolic stimulation. Meat is also rich in mitochondria, which contain all the essential nutrients for muscle tissue. It has been widely believed that veganism compromises the ability to naturally increase muscle mass.

However, by incorporating certain food combinations, including beans and nuts, vegans may reclaim their ability to materialize anabolic potential and induce muscular development. Nuts, especially almonds, have been considered an aphrodisiac food from the time of antiquity. With their superior nutritional content, almonds should be regarded as one of the most potent anabolic-supporting foods. Certain kinds of vegetarianism, such as lacto-vegetarianism (allowing consumption of dairy), can be a very effective diet. Dairy products such as whey cheese or yogurt made from cow, goat, sheep, or buffalo milk are excellent sources of protein rich in branch-chain amino acids. Whey protein, when processed correctly, is an excellent additional protein as well. Dairy should be organic and free of hormones, pesticides, and other adverse chemicals that affect muscularity, fat-burning, and overall health.

Conclusions: The Anabolic Cycle

- The first stage of the anabolic cycle is immediate but short and unstable.
- The second stage of the anabolic cycle's effect is delayed but can persist steadily for days.
- The body has limited peptide-stimulating and adrenal hormone reserves. Chronic activation of these hormones, such as from overtraining, can result in adrenal exhaustion, hormone insufficiency, and impaired ability to cope with stress or gain strength.
- Undereating combined with exercise is the best way to maximize the impact of the first stimulating stage of the anabolic cycle.

- Post-exercise recovery meals can help materialize an initial growth stimulation into actual growth.
- Overeating (or compensating) while providing the body with a full nutritional support that includes EFAs, complete protein, and sufficient fuel from carbs or fat will help finalize the anabolic cycle's second stage.
- Both omega-6 and omega-3 EFAs are necessary for completion of the anabolic cycle. Omega-6 is primarily a Stage I preliminary growth-stimulating agent. Omega-3, primarily a Stage II agent, is an anti-inflammatory that helps the body recuperate and build tissue.
- Both exercise and rest sessions are necessary for inducing a maximum anabolic state.

THE ANABOLIC CYCLE

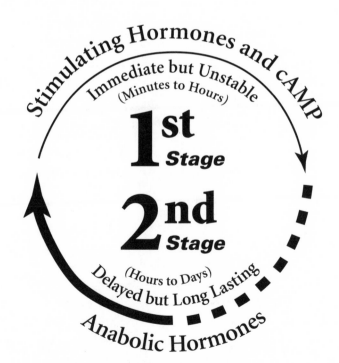

CHAPTER 8

Super Muscle: How to Develop Muscle with Superior Biological Capabilities

B uilding muscle demands skill, discipline, and experience, not to mention knowledge, instinct, logic, and certainly a degree of obsession. An obsessive commitment to endure pain in order to achieve the goal of physical excellence is one quality that has characterized athletes and warriors for thousands of years.

Obsession, however, sometimes means adhering to rigid routines that adversely affect performance. People who obsessively engage in long, exhausting exercise routines in an attempt to gain muscle mass often find themselves losing muscle instead. When this occurs, obviously it's a sign that something is wrong, but nevertheless it is common to see how obsessive individuals adamantly continue with their familiar routines, regardless of whether they're effective or not.

An athlete who wants to discover why his approach doesn't work must understand the real effects of various training methods on the muscle's capacity to perform. The following pages reveal facts about muscular development and address questions that are often overlooked. Revolutionary concepts are presented such as *muscle shifting* and how to develop a *super muscle* with superior biological capabilities.

Size and Power

Muscle size is only one of many factors that affect muscle performance. In fact big, heavy muscles sometimes compromise performance, particularly endurance and speed, as is often the case with long-distance runners or sprinters.

Muscle gain is likely part of a survival mechanism that helped humans gain strength via adaptation to stress. Survival is the most dominant driving force of life. The body will initiate any inherent mechanism needed to improve chances of survival, including muscle gain or even muscle waste. Survival depends on performance, and performance depends on more than just muscle size. From a survival point of view, what really counts is overall power.

"Power" is a term that is often confused with "strength." While we admire strength and size, we sometimes fail to understand that muscle size has only a limited correlation with muscle power. Power is the total sum of all performance capabilities, including strength, speed, velocity, endurance, and elasticity. In other words, muscle power is defined as the balance among all related performance capabilities:

- Strength—Resistance to weight load
- Velocity—Explosive impact (acceleration of force)
- Speed—Rhythm of repetitive moves per time (slow to fast)
- Endurance—Resistance to fatigue
- Elasticity—Stretched muscle resistance to breakdown (muscle resistance to tearing and injury)

All the above factors contribute to muscle power, although they may seem somewhat contradictory. For example, speed seems to antagonize strength, and strength seems to antagonize endurance. Apparently the rules of survival dictate priorities. For instance, if one needs to be fast, light, and mighty to survive, the body will develop lean muscles with high speed and velocity's explosive impact—such as we see with light-weight boxers or gymnasts.

On the other hand, strength gain requires exercise routines that maximize resistance and minimize endurance. Indeed, the common opinion among bodybuilders and powerlifters is that aerobics slows muscle gain. Moreover, anecdotal evidence suggests that muscle mass and strength gain require intense resistance exercise with a load of about eighty to ninety percent maximum voluntary contraction to be effective. For the purpose of strength and mass gain, performing sets of five to ten repetitions is recommended. In fact, it has been suggested that even one super-heavy set would be enough to stimulate muscle growth.

Nevertheless, because performance involves more than just muscle mass and strength, and because strength-specific training may compromise other performance capabilities such as speed and endurance, one may wonder whether the typical resistance training routines are effective enough to maximize performance, or for that matter improve survival. That question raises an issue of utmost importance for competitive athletes, martial artists, or even bodybuilders who seriously wish to break the conventional rules of sport conditioning (that improve a certain performance capability at the expense of others) and instead build a powerful body, superior in all performance capabilities.

Fast-Twitch and Slow-Twitch Muscles

Muscle fiber types are commonly classified as fast-twitch or slow-twitch. A fast-twitch fiber can generate more force, velocity, and speed than a slow fiber. Muscles with a high percentage of fast-twitch fibers are inherently stronger and faster than muscles consisting of mostly slow-twitch fibers. Most importantly, a fast-twitch fiber is capable of gaining more mass than a slow fiber.

For that reason, bodybuilders are usually interested in developing muscle with a high percentage of fast-twitch fiber to maximize muscle mass and strength gain. Considering all the advantages of fast-twitch fiber muscle, you might think that it is indeed superior to the slow-fiber type. Well, think again. From a biological point of view, slow-twitch fiber (also known as red fiber) can potentially outperform fast-twitch muscle fiber in several ways:

- Slow fibers are more resistant to fatigue.
- Slow fibers, with their higher mitochondrial content

(up to twenty percent of cellular volume), have superior metabolic capacity to utilize energy from fat fuel.

- Slow fibers have a high collagen content and are therefore more elastic and resistant to wear and tear.
- An increase in slow muscle fiber enhances vascularity and improves blood circulation as well as oxygenation.
- Finally, recent studies and experiments suggest that, from an evolutionary perspective, slow-twitch fiber Type I is more developed and advanced than fast-twitch fiber Type II.

Studies on muscle atrophy discovered that muscle retardation caused by prolonged misuse or injury involves the spontaneous conversion of the more developed slow fiber type into a more primitive type, the fast fiber. Surprise! As controversial as it may seem, from an evolutionary standpoint, developing big freaky muscles high in fast-twitch fiber may in fact be regarded as a sign of a biological setback.

Another element that needs to be examined is muscle capacity to generate energy. Survival depends on energy utilization. As noted, slow fiber, with its higher mitochondrial content, is much more efficient in converting fat to energy, a fact that contributes to a massive superiority in energy production, protection from insulin resistance, and an increase in fat mobilization to energy.

Nonetheless, fast fibers still can outperform slow fibers in strength, velocity, and speed, and human beings and animals need all physical performance capabilities to survive. Simply stated, both fast-twitch and slow-twitch fiber types are critically important for both short and prolonged actions.

Now, just when you believe you have a clear understanding of muscle fiber types, you will be confused all over again when further examining how all this relates to performance. Both speed and strength training target fast-twitch fiber. However, speed antagonizes strength, and vice versa. A race horse is built differently than a working horse; the same difference applies to athletes who train for speed versus those who train for strength. Most training methods today specifically target strength, or speed, or endurance, given that strength compromises endurance, endurance may compromise speed, and speed may compromise strength.

Considering all the above contradictions and variations, one may wonder whether it is possible to develop a super muscle that possesses all performance capabilities in one—muscle with superior strength, speed, velocity, and endurance capabilities, a "super muscle" with superior utilization and generation of energy.

Developing Super Muscles

The question of whether it is possible to build super muscle leads directly to the issue of muscle performance. When muscle superiority is the goal, maximum performance is the way. Muscular performance depends on two critical factors: (1) muscle composition and (2) nerve-to-muscle efficiency. More specifically, the type of muscle fiber and the efficiency of neural stimulation are the factors that dictate muscle performance and its potential to adapt and develop.

Muscle Wiring

To possess high-performance capabilities, a muscle must be composed of superior muscle fiber with superior neural wiring. The nervous system controls skeletal muscle through a network of neurons that are connected to muscle fibers via special junctions. A nerve can activate few or many fibers with either light or intense stimulation.

A nerve-to-muscle complex is called a neuro-motor unit. These can intermingle to facilitate compound muscle movement. All voluntary muscle actions originate in the brain. The more efficient the body's wiring is, the more intense the nervous stimulation can be, and the faster and more intensely the muscle can perform. Therefore, the definition of a super muscle clearly relates to its neural wiring.

Neuro-motor efficiency in the muscle increases via a process called innervation. As noted, the more wired the muscle is, the stronger and faster it becomes. Also, the more intense the stimulus is, the more anabolic the results will be. In fact, muscles that are wired with myelated neurons (the ones surrounded by myelin sheaths, which are isolated and can generate stronger neuro signals) are also muscles with substantial improved power and growth potential.

If there is indeed a super muscle, then it should have superior wiring, superior performance capabilities, and superior capacity to utilize energy. As to whether all this is possible—the answer is most likely, yes.

There is evidence that repetitive, intense stimulations signal the muscle to increase neuro-muscular efficiency via innervation. As noted, innervation is a process that increases or intensifies neural connections to muscle. It has also been suggested that this process by itself can significantly improve muscle strength or speed even without any change in muscle mass. However, different actions require different stimuli, with possibly different neuro-muscular adjustments.

In other words, to have superior performance capabilities, the muscle needs to be super-wired with a network of neural junctions that can help generate all specific performance capabilities, including strength, speed, velocity, and endurance. How to super-wire the muscle? That's a bit tricky. Again, muscle wiring is regulated via innervation. Muscle innervation can be improved through a repetitive complex of stimulatory signals that force adaptation and improvement. Change in exercise intensity is one way to signal adaptation, but the most profound way to force maximum improvement is by incorporating exercise of all performance capabilities (strength, speed, velocity, and endurance) in a single drill.

This is an intense and demanding training method. However, to be effective, this grueling combination of strength, speed, velocity, and endurance in a single drill must be repeated a few times per week. The repetitive complex of stimuli forces the muscle to adapt by increasing its neuro-wiring efficiency while improving all performance capabilities simultaneously.

The benefits can be astonishing. For instance, a long-distance runner with an inability to develop speed may be able to improve his sprinting capacity without compromising his overall endurance, consequently being able to break his or her own time record by facilitating a better sprint across the finish line.

Martial artists and boxers who already incorporate speed, velocity, and endurance in training may be able to gain additional strength on top of all this, and thereby improve power punches, push-pull movements, grappling, and overall resistance to fatigue under intense physical stress.

All that said, muscle neural wiring is only one part of what defines a super muscle.

We still need to acknowledge the most elemental unit of which the super muscle is composed: the *super muscle fiber.*

Super Muscle Fiber

Muscular development involves the conversion of one fiber type to another. It is generally accepted that short, intense resistance exercise routines are likely to increase the conversion of slow-twitch Type I fibers into fast-twitch Type II fibers. Conversely, long, repetitive, low-impact aerobic training routines are likely to increase the conversion of fast-twitch fiber types into slower ones.

These conversions of muscle fiber serve an obvious biological purpose. Stated simply, the body adapts to the most intense or long-lasting stimuli by changing the composition of its muscle fibers accordingly. Moreover, the signal for muscular development occurs instantly. When stimulated by the neurotransmitter acetylcholine, the muscle reverses its electrical charge and establishes a cellular state called "action potential." This process involves a cascade of events including the induction of ion channels and the production of certain proteins and enzymes that initiate muscle contraction and also signal growth potential.

Much is still unknown about exactly how muscular development occurs. Nevertheless, based on animal and human studies, researchers suggest that muscular development most likely has to do with repetitive stimulation and actions that encode gene transcriptions, which signal protein synthesis and growth, presumably via activation of the calcium channel that regulates the concentration of calcium ions in the cell. Every moment of action starts a process that, with a repetitive amplifying effect, can potentially lead to muscle transformation. Considering that fast fibers have short endurance, whereas slow fibers are weak and slow, you might wonder what muscular development really means. Can you ever be in a win-win situation in which you gain both strength and endurance?

Since human survival inherently depends on all performance capabilities, including strength, speed, and endurance, it is reasonable to assume that there is a biological mechanism within us that is primarily programmed for improving survival skills by maximizing overall power impact through increasing all of these capabilities together. Evidence suggests that there is indeed a biological mechanism that under certain conditions will develop a superior muscle fiber that can outperform any other muscle fiber type.

The so-called "super muscle" fiber carries all possible performance-related advantages. Scientists have already found a kind of super muscle fiber high in both mitochondrial enzymes and glycolytic enzymes, a combination that can afford superiority in both prolonged aerobic exercise and short, intense, anaerobic exercise. Note that conventional muscle fibers are either high in mitochondrial enzymes but low in glycolytic enzymes (slow fibers) or vice versa (fast fibers), a fact that limits their capacity to utilize fuel. In any case, super muscle fibers are somehow classified as part of the family of fast Type II fibers, albeit with superior endurance capabilities similar to those of slow Type I fibers. That classification, however, may be misleading. The unique structure and biological functions of the super fibers should make them a distinct type of muscle fiber with unique cellular composition and ultra-superior performance capabilities.

The percentage of super fibers in an average human muscle today is almost negligible. Current sport-specific conditioning and exercise programs, based on isolation of body parts as well as separation between strength, speed, velocity, and endurance, most likely fail to trigger the biological mechanism that improves overall power impact, thereby diminishing the chance of developing super muscle fibers.

Like other wild apes, such as gorillas and chimpanzees, our ancestors most probably carried significantly higher percentages of super muscle fibers than we do today. Humans frequently were engaged in fight or flight activities that incorporated speed, endurance, and strength—all of which are required for human survival and therefore are inherently programmed in each of us.

To develop super muscle fibers, you will need to adjust your workout routines to incorporate special exercise drills that include strength, speed, velocity, and endurance all in one. For instance, you can incorporate a giant superset that consists of sprint intervals, clean presses, chin-ups, and heavy bag punching. Minimize rest time between sets. If you are a martial artist, try to incorporate repetitive sets of combined strength and explosive exercise into your routines, such as with shoulder presses followed immediately by a set of fast, explosive punches. If you aren't a competitive athlete, you can still incorporate super muscle training.

Slow-motion moves such as those of Tai Chi or Qigong can efficiently increase power-punch-explosive impact. The slow moves signal strength stimuli, whereas the fast moves signal speed and velocity. In combination, slow and fast actions—as we get with a combination of strength and speed exercise—will signal the muscle to improve its speed, explosiveness, and overall power impact.

Boxers and martial artists often lack the ability to generate a knockout punch. Ideally this information can help them develop muscle fibers with improved neural wiring and increased capacity to deliver and endure explosive and intense performance with max power-punch impact even in late rounds.

This is an extreme training method that, if overdone, may lead to overtraining, so remember: keep your workout short.

Start by incorporating one super-muscle workout per week in your regular training routine, and build up gradually. Adjust the workout according to your specific priorities, with the goal of strengthening weaknesses while integrating strength, speed, velocity, and endurance, all together. Be patient. The threshold time for actual adaptation can last up to a few weeks.

Finally, nutrition is critical for your progress. Proper application of recovery meals consisting of chemical-free quality proteins and slow-releasing carbs is necessary to facilitate fast recuperation, inhibit muscle breakdown, and maximize growth potential after exercise. You can find more information on super muscle training at www.warriordiet.com (under CFT).

Muscle Shifting: Improving Body Proportion

The failure to reach peak performance is sometimes the result of dysfunctional body proportion. When the body's natural symmetry is interrupted due to incorrect training, injuries, or aging, some body parts can grow disproportionately to others. As a result, the oversized body parts assume most of the body's workload, rendering the undeveloped parts prone to further inactivity and resulting degradation. If uncorrected, unbalanced body proportions may lead to a vicious cycle in which the strong body part gets stronger and larger while the weak body part gets weaker and smaller.

Unfortunately, this problem is commonly overlooked. Large-chested men often do multiple sets of bench presses while chronically neglecting their legs. There are also those "two-dimensional guys" who work only the body parts they see in the mirror. Two-dimensional people often carry a big chest and biceps but have a flat back and buttocks.

Typical workout routines are not sufficient to reverse body deformations and establish new body proportions. Hell, they often make it worse. Body disproportions seem to be a curse—is there anything that can be done to reverse it? Well, there is, but this is something that may again go against anything you've read or heard. I'm referring to a process that can force the body to redesign itself and create new, improved body proportions with improved performance capabilities. This process is called *muscle shifting*. To understand how it is possible to improve body proportion, you need to acquaint yourself with the biological mechanism that regulates muscle gain and muscle waste.

Muscle Gain versus Muscle Waste

Muscle gain is a process by which muscle adds more protein to its mass than it loses. Gain and loss of muscle protein is part of a regulatory mechanism that helps the body constantly maintain homeostasis of its protein pool. Protein is needed for numerous critical metabolic functions, including the production of enzymes and hormones, formation of antibodies, and repair of old and broken tissue. For this reason, maintaining a protein pool is of the utmost importance for survival. Skeletal muscles serve as the body's exclusive protein storage organs. Proteins are synthesized or degraded according to the body's specific needs. For instance, injuries, disease, or prolonged starvation increase the body's demand for protein and therefore are often associated with protein degradation and muscle wasting.

A healthy, 160-pound male has a daily protein turnover of about 280–300 grams. "Protein turnover" is a term that describes the total amount of protein consumed and utilized for anabolic and catabolic purposes. Muscle gain clearly depends on the rate of protein turnover, in particular on the rates of protein synthesis versus protein degradation. In fact, any process that induces muscle gain also involves a surplus of protein synthesis over protein breakdown.

Actual muscle mass gain clearly depends on two critically important processes: the first promotes a gain in muscle protein, and the second inhibits muscle waste. Anything that helps inhibit muscle waste effectively promotes muscle gain, a fact that is often overlooked.

Since carbohydrates are commonly considered "bad guys" among dieters and fitness advocates, many active individuals who wish to sustain a lean body tend to restrict carb consumption, not realizing that by doing so they severely compromise their opportunity to effectively build muscle. Insulin, among other functions, is an anti-catabolic hormone that by any means inhibits muscle breakdown. That's why it is so important to incorporate small recovery meals that contain both protein and carbs after exercise. The anti-catabolic, anti-muscle-waste effect of insulin also explains why a state of insulin resistance or diabetes is often associated with muscle waste.

Other factors that help prevent muscle waste include anabolic hormones, inhibition of stress hormones, and the ingestion of dietary protein, especially branch-chain amino acids (BCAA). The amino acid leucine (in BCAA) has a profound inhibitory effect on muscle protein degradation. This is also true for the actions of anabolic agents such as growth hormone, testosterone, IGF1, and its related heat-shock protein 27, all of which increase muscle protein conservation, thereby inhibiting muscle waste.

Incorporating special dietary and training methods that reduce stress can effectively suppress cortisol's catabolic effect on muscle protein.

Relaxation and proper rest intervals are as important as exercise, and avoiding overtraining is also important. Overtraining may lead to stagnation, plateau, hormonal decline, and loss of muscle tissue.

Let Your Body Redesign Itself

Most protein synthesis originates from endogenous sources, not from dietary sources. This suggests that muscle gain is actually a process of recycling in which the body converts endogenous protein into new muscle fibers. It also leads to the startling conclusion that the body can, in fact, redesign itself by shifting protein from one body part to another.

Under certain conditions that involve intense physical stress and a low protein intake, the body will try to sustain performance and improve its conditioning by changing its muscular proportions, shifting protein from less active muscles to more active muscles, thereby creating a more adjusted and functional body proportion. Note that protein shifting is a natural process that occurs every time you fast or undereat and will be further accelerated if you also exercise. Recycling old tissue into new tissue is an inherent healing method that helps maintain tissue integrity and slow age-related wear and tear. This awesome process is all but inhibited by chronic feeding.

The question that arises is how can you signal your body to redesign itself? You may be able to do it in the following way: First, exercise targeting mostly the body parts that you wish to build, while minimizing work on the overgrown body parts. Second, alternate between days of low protein intake and days of moderate to high protein intake. This dietary method, combined with exercise that targets and prioritizes certain muscles, will likely trigger the recycling process that shifts protein from one muscle to another—from the non-active one to the active one—thereby helping you design new body proportions.

Preservation of Active Muscles

Evidence demonstrates that a low-protein diet with sufficient calories triggers a mechanism that inhibits active muscle breakdown.[5] That mechanism presumably helps the body survive under conditions of low protein intake by sparing active muscles' protein from degradation. It is possible, then, that a temporary low-protein diet combined with exercise will force the body to mobilize protein in one direction only—from less active muscles to more active muscles, thus sparing the more active muscles while using the less active ones as an endogenous source of protein.

This process will naturally redesign the body to be more functional. If you want to improve your body proportions, you may find this method well worth trying. In any case, try workout routines that incorporate strength, speed, and endurance exercise all together. This will enhance not just the induction of body transformation, but also improve overall performance.

Muscle shifting is a new term derived from an old concept. The idea of shifting muscles is based on the body's tendency to adapt and improve its functionality by strengthening those muscles responsible for actions that occur most and are most intense.

Again, a person may be able to shift muscles by establishing special workout sessions five to six times per week that prioritize certain body parts (those that need extra strengthening) while maintaining other body parts (those that are either overgrown or relatively overpowering and need to be reduced in size). As noted, cycling between days of low and high protein consumption is a safe way to help the body redesign itself. Low-protein days are likely to trigger the mechanism that inhibits active muscle breakdown, thereby forcing the body to dig into its protein pool from less active muscles, shifting protein from them to the more active muscles. This process will maintain and increase the size of active muscles while gradually decreasing the size of less active muscles.

Following this, on high-protein days, the body will take advantage of a window of opportunity to maximize protein utilization after low-protein days. Following a low protein intake, there is a substantial increase in the capacity to utilize protein (most likely a compensation mechanism). This can result in overall increased muscle mass.

In conclusion, muscle shifting—the process that facilitates protein shifting from one muscle to another—can potentially help individuals correct body proportion and symmetry, thereby improving both aesthetics and performance.

Muscle Nourishment

Instant muscle gain is the main motto upon which fitness and body-building ad campaigns are based. Companies that sell nutritional supplements and powdered protein products often promise a quick fix to anyone who uses their products. Commercial sport nutrition companies are clearly taking advantage of people's willingness to believe the unbelievable. Consequently, tons of powdered protein and "miracle pills" are purchased and consumed daily by people hoping for immediate muscle gain.

Interestingly, commercial protein powders and dry pet food are packed in very similar containers—the only difference is that pet food products are generally superior to sport nutrition products. In fact, if you ever try to serve your pet a commercial protein shake, you'll realize that cats and dogs hate the smell and taste of human powdered-protein products. Animals know better. They hate the strong chemical odor, artificial additives, and sweeteners, as well as the degraded, cheap, and over-processed proteins that are typically found in sport nutrition and diet products. Regardless of whether human protein products are graded below the standard suitable for animal consumption, there is no doubt that muscle nourishment must come from chemical-free and minimally processed sources. Muscular development is an issue that goes far beyond just pumping iron and shoving protein. In fact, incorrect pumping and cheap-quality protein may adversely affect overall metabolism and impair muscle gain.

The principle of muscle nourishment is *complete nutrition in sufficient amounts.* In other words, all essential nutrients and fuel needed—including vitamins, minerals, antioxidants, probiotics, EFAs, essential amino acids, carbs, fat, and fiber—must be consumed in sufficient amounts to afford a complete recuperation and muscular development.

Carbs, even though not technically essential, should be regarded as conditionally essential food for muscles because of their profound anti-catabolic effect on muscle breakdown as well as the enhancement of insulin's anabolic actions on the muscles. Proteins should always come from whole-food sources. Animal and marine foods such as eggs, fish, and other seafood are the best sources of complete protein. Dairy foods, particularly yogurt, cheese, and whey protein, are rich in branch-chain amino acids and immuno-supportive globulins, which help inhibit muscle protein breakdown and promote fast recuperation.

It is also critically important to ingest sufficient amounts of protein and avoid chronic low-protein diets. Protein deficiencies force the body to break down muscle protein for other metabolic purposes, thereby causing undesirable muscle waste. Just as important as proteins are the essential fatty acids, whose anabolic actions are major contributors to the overall growth impact.

Finally, vitamins, minerals, and antioxidants are necessary to catalyze all cellular functions including energy production and to prevent a metabolic shutdown. Antioxidants help neutralize toxins and accelerate the removal of inflammatory compounds that otherwise would inhibit recuperation and muscular development. Active individuals need to consume more nutritional supplements (from natural, chemical-free sources) than people who don't exercise to satisfy their body's increased demand for all the above essential nutrients.

Post-Exercise Recovery Meals

The importance of recovery meals is often overlooked or misunderstood, yet knowing how and when to incorporate a recovery meal can make a difference in strength and muscularity gains. Post-exercise recovery meals serve two major functions:

1. They promote actual growth by finalizing the actions of all anabolic agents, including growth hormone, IGF1, testosterone, and insulin.
2. They prevent muscle breakdown, enhance recuperation, and materialize growth.

An effective recovery lies in the beginning of the recuperation process. Right after the workout, there is a period lasting from thirty minutes up to four hours, known as *the post-exercise window of opportunity*. That's when the body's growth-promoting hormones reach peak levels, when insulin reaches peak sensitivity, and precisely when recovery meals should be ingested. At this time the muscle has its highest potential to assimilate nutrients, recuperate, and develop (by increasing protein utilization in the muscle). Timing is critical. The capacity of any meal to promote recuperation and muscular development relates to the following formula:

Right nutrition at the right time equals maximum recuperation and facilitation of muscular development. In other words: "It's when you eat that makes what you eat matter." Note that taking advantage of increased insulin sensitivity may be one of the key elements in designing recovery meals after strenuous resistance training.

[As a little background, it has been established that this post-exercise period is characterized by improved insulin sensitivity. Many studies have indicated that both endurance and resistance training increase insulin sensitivity.]

To actually promote an immediate recuperating effect, a recovery meal should take full advantage of the window of opportunity and theoretically be ingested during the first thirty minutes, right after intense exercise. Nevertheless, after prolonged intense drills it is recommended that one wait thirty minutes up to an hour before ingesting a recovery meal. The reason: prolonged intense drills cause an accumulation of lactic acid in the muscles and the liver, which leads to a temporary state of insulin resistance. This waiting period lets the body clear the lactic acid, regain insulin sensitivity, and then have a recovery meal. Any further delay in the timing of the recovery meal may attenuate its full beneficial effect on the muscle and the recuperation process.

A post-exercise recovery meal should provide a blend of fast-releasing nutrients as well as slow-releasing nutrients required for promoting both short-term and long-term muscle hypertrophy. The following nutrients are needed:

- **Protein with maximum biological value containing a blend of fast- and slow-releasing proteins,** such as whey combined with milk protein. Amount per serving should be between 10 and 30g (depending on training intensity and volume). The fast-releasing proteins will help boost an immediate post-exercise protein synthesis, whereas the slow-releasing proteins will help sustain the already established anabolic state in the muscle tissue.

- **Carbohydrates consisting of a blend of fast- and slow-releasing carbs,** specially designed for inducing an optimum insulin spike, followed by a steady, slow carb release required for stabilizing insulin levels as well as maintaining an optimum level of blood sugar. Moderate amounts of post-exercise fast-releasing carbs (fructose-free simple carbs) should immediately inhibit muscle protein breakdown without over-spiking insulin. Then the slow-releasing carbs (complex or fibrous carbs) will help maintain this anti-catabolic activity in the muscle tissue for a longer period of time (depending on amount of carbs ingested). Quantities should be between 10 and 30g. Most of the carbs should come from a low-glycemic complex fibrous source to avoid over-spiking insulin and experiencing undesirable blood sugar fluctuations. However, a small amount of simple carbs from natural low-glycemic sources, preferably fructose-free such as rice, malt, or maple syrup, may help induce a short-term insulin spike required to facilitate an immediate post-exercise anti-catabolic effect. Five grams of simple carbs will do the job. As noted, any excess of sugar may cause insulin fluctuations, hypoglycemia, and undesirable inhibition of fat loss.

    Post-exercise carb ingestion also helps promote swift IGF1 actions in the muscles, increased levels of which are believed to be the most immediate factor in muscle hypertrophy.

- **Food Containing IGF1.** As mentioned, an increased IGF1 level in the muscle tissue is one of the most influential determinants in muscle hypertrophy. Therefore, having food naturally high in IGF1 such as whey or colostrum (a mammalian pre-milk) may be exactly what the body needs to induce maximum anabolic actions right after a workout. Some individuals may be sensitive to bovine dairy, due to high levels of certain proteins (betalactoglobulins). In that case, it may be worth trying fresh dairy products from other sources such as goat, sheep, or buffalo.

Whole goat or buffalo ricotta cheeses could be great sources of protein and IGF1. Food rich in IGF1 provides additional benefits. Both whey protein and colostrum help enhance recovery by virtue of their highly potent immuno-supporting globulins and related compounds. These are the same dairy proteins and immuno-supportive compounds commonly found in breast milk that help protect a newborn against infection or disease, and they will most likely provide similar benefits to an adult engaged in intense or prolonged strenuous exercise.

- **Good Fat.** To support immediate and long-term anabolic actions, a recovery meal requires good fat. However, only certain kinds of fat could be truly beneficial. The best oils for immediate recovery are energy-producing ergogenic oils such as MCT (medium-chain triglycerides) from natural coconut oil, which have been shown to convert to energy rather than body fat, or omega-9 monounsaturated fats such as those in nuts, seeds, and olive oil. Naturally occurring fat in dairy protein is rich in IGF1 and therefore beneficial.

  EFA n-3, also known as Omega 3 EFA (n-3), is obviously important by virtue of being both essential and anti-inflammatory. Nonetheless, n-3 can be added to the evening meal and doesn't need to be applied right after exercise. N-3 EFAs and monounsaturated oils help promote anti-inflammatory actions as well as steroid hormone actions. Furthermore, fat slows the release of carbs and serves as a nutritional cofactor in supporting protein utilization in the muscle.

  There are also special functional oils such as lecithin that help enhance liver functions and provide nutrients for the synthesis of the brain-to-muscle neurotransmitter acetylcholine. Lecithin also supports the muscle's increased demand for phosphates after intense exercise.

  Note: Stay away from rancid or hydrogenated oils, as well as omega-6 vegetable oils such as canola, corn, safflower, or soy, which in excess have been shown to promote estrogen, suppress recovery, and cause fat gain.

Summary

Have a recovery meal within thirty minutes up to an hour after your workout, to grant immediate post-exercise anabolic and anti-catabolic effects.

Recovery meals should ideally incorporate a blend of fast- and slow-releasing proteins and carbs, as well as good fat to support immediate and long-lasting anabolic actions.

Most importantly, a viable recovery meal should always comply with the following parameters: *all-natural, low-glycemic, great taste.* If one of these parameters is compromised, the recovery meal will not be viable. For instance, a funky aftertaste is a sign of chemicals, and an overly sweet taste is a sign of excessive sugar, both of which are detrimental to the viability of the meal and may harm the body's capacity to recuperate rather than supporting it.

Post-exercise recovery meals should be practical, handy, and readily available right after the workout.

To further promote an actual anabolic impact, the protein component of the meal should be made from a complete protein source naturally rich in immuno-supporting compounds and other nutritional cofactors including naturally occurring vitamins and minerals as well as beneficial fat.

Recovery meals should be made from either fresh, light, and fast-assimilating protein foods such as yogurt or kefir, or from specially designed all-natural, low-glycemic protein products (e.g. shakes or bars).

Avoid commercial products made with cheap isolated proteins, particularly soy, or products drenched with chemical preservatives, sugar, alcohol, and artificial sweeteners.

The following are examples of good post-exercise recovery meals.

Berries and yogurt (8 to 16 oz.). Combine 1 teaspoon of *colostrum* with yogurt or with a serving of protein shake containing fast- and slow-releasing proteins (such as whey and milk proteins), naturally supported with slow-releasing carbs and naturally sweetened.

Have a *protein shake or a protein bar* specially designed for recovery made with all-natural ingredients consisting of a blend of fast- and slow-releasing proteins derived from whey and milk as well as fast- and slow-releasing carbs (such as rice or malt syrup, oat bran, or rice bran). It should also contain good functional fat, preferably with minimum capacity to convert into body fat (such as MCT oil or lecithin).

Again, protein shakes and bars could be very useful and handy as post-exercise *recovery meals,* provided that they are free of chemical preservatives, sugar, alcohol, artificial sweeteners, hydrogenated oils, or toxins that may adversely suppress recovery, recuperation, and growth.

To support and help continue the anabolic effect of exercise, it is highly recommended to incorporate a few small recovery meals every 1–2 hours following the initial post-exercise recovery meal. These small recovery meals are critically important, particularly for those who work out early in the morning. Nevertheless, in order to avoid undesirable fat gain, reduce the carb component of the meals, starting with the second recovery meal.

For instance, those who work out in the morning should have a recovery meal with carbs right after the workout to induce an immediate anti-catabolic effect via insulin activity. Following that initial post-exercise recovery meal shake or bar, it is advisable to incorporate small protein meals (15–25g of protein with minimum carbs), such as plain yogurt, cheese, eggs, or all-natural low-carb no-sugar-added protein shake, every couple of hours to keep maintaining protein synthesis in the muscle tissues without adverse side effects. That way, one will be able to maintain high insulin sensitivity toward the end of the day enjoying eating big nightly meals while taking advantage of insulin's anabolic effect with a minimum risk of side effects.

The purpose of recovery meals is to nourish the starving muscles with maximum nutrition from minimum food, just enough to do the job. Recovery meals should therefore be carefully designed. Protein and other ingredients should be derived from high-quality, all-natural, and minimally processed sources.

Notice that carbohydrate meals and their related insulin spikes suppress GH secretion, but here is the trick: even though insulin initially suppresses GH secretion before exercise, it plays a critical role in actually finalizing the actions of both GH and IGF1 *after* exercise. In other words, post-exercise carb ingestion (with its accompanying insulin spike) is not only optimum but necessary for effectively promoting IGF1 actions in the muscle.

Knowing how and in particular when to incorporate meals can make the difference between a plateau and progress. If you have been doing everything "by the book" and are still failing to improve muscularity and strength, it is very likely that a good recovery meal is your missing link.

Some Practical Dietary Tips for Muscle Gain

- Commercial isolated and over-processed protein powders are often missing certain amino acids such as lysine and methionine and thus may result in imbalance and amino acid deficiencies. The body translates such an imbalance as a surplus of certain amino acids over the deficient ones. This forces the body to waste the "extra" amino acids in a desperate attempt to reach an optimum balance. Biological balance of essential amino acids is required for optimum cellular functions. The wasting of amino acids increases the metabolic stress on the body with toxic byproducts, all of which may lead to muscle wasting.
- As noted, ingestion of post-exercise carbs facilitates insulin actions that are critically important for the materialization of actual growth. Carbs should be derived from a fibrous starch or from fructose-free, relatively low-glycemic sweeteners such as rice or malt syrup.
- Minerals, especially calcium, magnesium, potassium, and zinc, as well as trace minerals such as chromium, molybdenum, and selenium, are highly recommended as post-exercise nutritional supplements. Minerals are necessary for all metabolic pathways and stress management. Minerals can be quickly depleted during physical activity. A post-exercise mineral deficiency can

lead to muscle cramps, headaches, and symptoms that resemble those of overtraining, including insomnia, nervousness, and exhaustion. Ideally, minerals should be supplemented every day.

- Minimize all chemical ingredients, including artificial sweeteners, sugar, alcohol, and chemical preservatives (including sulfites). All of these place immense metabolic stress on the liver. An overwhelmed liver may not be able to perform some of its critical duties, including the removal of toxins, the utilization of fat and carbs, and the metabolism of steroid hormones. This can lead to impaired energy utilization, insulin resistance, hormonal imbalance, and estrogenic reactions with symptoms including fat gain (in the belly and other stubborn-fat areas), feminization of men, and stunted growth.

- Make all your meals, including your recovery meals, appealing and tasty. There is evidence that taste and aroma correlate with the assimilation of nutrients and the sense of satiety. People who work hard to gain muscle should be wise enough to cultivate their sense of taste. Your body, your mind, and your palate all deserve full compensation for your hard work.

- People can opt to have light protein and a small amount of carbs just before a workout. A pre-workout meal should be designed to give the body just enough energy to initiate the workout. Pre-workout meals should operate on the same principles as a car or truck ignition. For instance, low-glycemic fruits such as berries, nonfat yogurt, or even a single shot of espresso are good to jump-start your engine.

Dietary cycles based on pumping and depleting carbs force the body to increase glycogen reserves and improve utilization of carbs for energy. These improvements in muscle fueling will pay generously during conditions that involve prolonged intense (nonaerobic) strength, speed, or velocity drills.

Carb depletion followed by carb-loading is a traditional method of increasing glycogen reserves in muscles, commonly used by long-distance runners. Nevertheless, it is important to note that it is the fast-twitch fibers that have a greater affinity for building glycogen reserves as an energy source for nonaerobic resistance exercise.

On the other hand, it is the slow-twitch fibers, with their larger mitochondrial capacity, that have a greater affinity for fat utilization for prolonged aerobic endurance training. Repeating patterns of feeding cycles that involve carb-loading days followed by fat-loading days would force the body to improve carb and fat utilization by increasing both glycogen reserves and mitochondrial capacity, with their respective enzymes.

For athletic purposes, it is important to distinguish between the effects of carb fuel and fat fuel on muscle performance. Carbs should be regarded mainly as food for fast fibers' nonaerobic actions, thereby enhancing strength, speed, and velocity, whereas fat should be regarded mostly as food for slow fibers' aerobic actions, thereby enhancing prolonged resistance to fatigue (endurance).

Incorporating high-carb and high-fat days with exercise will most likely improve all performance capabilities, increasing glycogen reserves and mitochondrial density for superior energy utilization. Note that days of high carbs should be low in fat, whereas days of high fat should be low in carbs. That way, one can enhance the effect of pumping and depleting each of these fuels. Note that similar patterns of feeding have been shown to significantly affect the body's adaptation to the most dominant fuel food. People who live primarily in freezing Arctic climates and consume mostly fatty marine foods are better adapted to fat utilization than people who live in warm climates whose primary fuel comes from plants and grain. It follows then that by the same logic, prolonged high-fat or high-carb diets can distinctively affect muscle fueling and performance.

The best dietary sources of carbohydrates are grains, plants, and roots.

The best dietary sources of fats—omega-6, omega-3, and omega-9—are nuts, seeds, marine food, avocados, and olive oil. Other oils such as sesame, grapeseed, and rice bran are also great sources of fatty acids and other cofactors including vitamins, antioxidants, and phytosterols. Repetitive cycles of carb-loading and fat-loading over prolonged periods, combined with the previously presented super muscle training program, have the potential to enhance the magnitude of physical transformation.

PART III

Fat Loss

M ost people in the United States are overweight. Thirty percent of the adult population is obese, with a fifty-percent obesity rate among people over fifty years of age. The rate of child obesity more than tripled from 1980 to 2004 and so did the rates of obesity among adolescents.[6] The rates of obesity in our society have been growing persistently. We're a nation becoming fatter and fatter, in spite of the ever-growing number of diet programs and products, gym memberships, weight loss pills, miracle cures, certified nutritionists, and billions of dollars spent annually on health care. Apparently, fat loss is not a simple issue. The fact is that, statistically, all fat-loss programs are failing miserably.

People who initially lose weight will gain it all back, and even more in the long run. Dieters often confuse fat loss with weight loss, but the two are very different processes. Fat loss is the process that leads to weight loss, and not the other way around.

Of special concern is stubborn fat, the tenacious fat tissue known to be almost impossible to get rid of. Stubborn fat generally resists fat-burning actions and can't be removed even by hard diet and exercise. Stubborn fat gain is a modern problem of almost epidemic proportions. Both men and women of all age groups suffer from the inability to lose stubborn fat, primarily because they have limited information about it and are poorly equipped to tackle the problem.

The subject of fat loss gets even more complicated for physically active people. In spite of hard training and strict diet routines, many active individuals are struggling to lose excess fat with no results. Eager to be lean 'n' mean or at the top of one's sport, competitive and highly active men and women often resort to extreme diets that shatter their metabolism, resulting in fatigue, loss of libido, loss of strength, and vulnerability to disease.

With the continued lack of definitive guidelines for weight loss, the question still exists: *how to lose body fat and stay lean?*

The only way to effectively address this question, including how to eliminate stubborn fat, is to first understand the biological basis of fat metabolism—how and why fat gain or fat loss occurs. When you understand this, you will realize that fat tissue enables functions besides simply providing a storage site for energy. Fat tissue serves distinct purposes that give it reasons to accumulate, protecting the body from the adverse effects of certain metabolic disorders by inducing fat gain.

The biological principle of fat loss is very simple: Removing the responsibilities of fat tissue will remove the reasons for its existence. By doing so, one can lose body fat with astonishing efficiency and, most importantly, stay lean for life.

CHAPTER 9

The Biological Principles of Fat Loss

F at loss is part of a biological process that forces the body to break storage fat and release fatty acid for energy. But simple as it may sound, fat-burning isn't just about turning fat to energy. In fact, the burning of fat, including stubborn fat, requires some preliminary steps that have nothing to do with fat-burning *per se*. To effectively break fat-storing cells for energy, one must first eliminate the very reasons for fat gain. This way, it's possible to establish the right metabolic environment that favors conversion of fat to energy. There is growing evidence that certain metabolic impairments such as high toxicity, insulin resistance, and hormonal imbalance give fat tissue a reason to accumulate and resist elimination.

It is commonly believed that fat tissues serve as storage for energy. But it's a less well-known fact that adipose (fat) tissues also serve other biological purposes. The body gains or loses fat as part of a regulatory mechanism that helps protect it from three major problems:

1. *Accumulation of toxins that can damage vital organs.*
2. *Accumulation of lipids and cholesterol that can lead to insulin resistance and diabetes.*
3. *Hormonal imbalance such as imbalance of androgens and estrogens in men and women, respectively.*

Hormonal imbalance can lead to an array of metabolic problems, including loss of bone mass, cognitive difficulties, impaired sexual performance, and accelerated aging. In other words, fat gain can be regarded as a desperate attempt by the body to protect itself from high levels of toxins, insulin resistance (or diabetes), and imbalance of hormones. Therefore any method that will help eliminate the three problems cited above would likely remove the three most influential reasons for fat gain—thereby breaking fat-loss plateaus while facilitating a notable leaning-down effect. Let's examine how different approaches affect fat loss.

Carbohydrate and Calorie Restrictions

Most current diets are based on two major premises: (1) restriction of calories and (2) restriction of carbohydrates (carbs). Fat-restrictive diets were popular a couple of decades ago but failed to help people lose weight. They're still viable today for treating cardiovascular disorders. By restricting calories, the body consumes less energy than it spends; therefore it is theoretically forced to burn stored fat to provide the required missing energy. In a similar way, carbohydrate restriction forces the body to burn fat instead.

Additionally, carb and calorie restrictions have been shown to lower insulin and, for that matter, minimize its inhibitory effects on fat-burning.

Yet in spite of the convincing logic behind the above premises, neither calorie nor carb restrictions are sufficient to sustain fat loss over the long run. Something else must be going on. For thousands of years, people living in China, Tibet, and Africa have been following diets traditionally based on grains and roots. Yet in spite of consuming high-carb meals, these people stay leaner than people living in the U.S.—even considering the ever-growing number of dieters among American people. There are also societies of people who traditionally consume huge quantities of food, such as the nomadic Arab tribes in the North African and Middle Eastern deserts. These people are famous for their huge feasts, yet their bodies typically look as rugged as the desert rocks.

Chronic restriction of calories and carbs actually can be counter-effective (cause the opposite effect): even though people initially lose some weight, they typically gain it all back and even more. These restrictions have been shown to shatter the thyroid hormone and inhibit sex hormones, leading to a sluggish metabolism with a suppressed libido, and diminished ability to lose fat. All that said, calorie and carb restrictions, *if managed properly,* can actually be highly beneficial in promoting long-term fat loss. If done periodically rather than chronically, restricting calories and carbs can be a very effective method for helping people lose body fat and even stay lean.

Fat loss is a topic that requires further investigation. There is an urgent need for information regarding the various biological functions for which fat is responsible. There is also a need for practical methods that can help remove the biological functions (or obstacles) that give fat a reason to accumulate. When fat is deprived of its active role, it loses its biological function and, like any other dysfunctional organ, it degrades and decreases in size.

Similar to muscle, fat can either be built or destroyed. The body's survival depends on its tendency to develop active tissue and degrade inactive tissue. The same holds true for fat. Deprive fat of its active role, and it will break down and shrink.

Eliminating the Reasons for Fat to Exist

Eliminating the reasons for the accumulation of fat is a mission that, at first glance, looks impossible. A certain amount of body fat is necessary for survival, and therefore the idea of completely eliminating body fat is implausible. Nevertheless, by eliminating the metabolic reason(s) behind fat gain, it will be possible to effectively reduce body fat to a minimum biological set point at which the body still performs at its best. To do this, we must first examine the two distinct types of fat tissue: subcutaneous and visceral.

Subcutaneous and Visceral Fat

One of the main reasons for confusion about fat loss is that many people aren't aware that there are two kinds of fat tissue in the body, each with a distinct sensitivity to fat breakdown, or lipolysis. These two distinct fat tissues are *subcutaneous fat,* which lies under the skin, and *visceral fat,* which is internal.

Subcutaneous fat tends to be insulin-sensitive and therefore more resistant to fat-burning, whereas visceral fat is more insulin-resistant and has a higher affinity for adrenal fat-burning stimulation than sub-cutaneous fat. Nonetheless, both types of fat tissues somehow balance the breakdown of each other.

For instance, the greater the amount of visceral fat (such as in the belly area), the more it releases fatty acids and the more resistant to fat-burning subcutaneous fat will be. Because of its rapid reaction to adre-nal stimulation followed by fat breakdown and the release of fatty acids to the liver, visceral fat is presumably most dangerous to individuals who are prone to cardiovascular disease or diabetes. High visceral fat and its related flux of released fatty acids may cause fatty liver (hepatic hyperlipidemia) and consequent insulin resistance and hypertension.

The accumulation of visceral fat is often associated with the forma-tion of stubborn fat under the skin. In an attempt to balance visceral fat's high release of fatty acids to the liver, the subcutaneous fat tends to be more resistant to fat-burning and in turn becomes stubborn.

Delayed Fat Loss

Another reason for confusion about fat loss is the often-delayed manner in which fat loss occurs. People who suffer from accumulation of exces-sive visceral fat often don't see any noticeable reduction of subcutaneous fat, in spite of following hard diet and exercise routines. The reason is that visceral fat responds first to the fat-burning stimulation of diet and exercise, whereas subcutaneous fat has a delayed reaction. People with large amounts of visceral fat need to first get rid of its excess before notic-ing any reduction in the fat under the skin. Individuals who want to reach a lean and defined muscularity must be aware that the higher a person's percentage of visceral fat, the more he or she will suffer from delayed fat loss and the longer it will take to notice a change in body composition and muscle definition.

Fat Functions

Researchers believe that fat metabolism is controlled by inherent biological mechanisms that help humans survive in extreme conditions such as starvation, cold climates, or exposure to prolonged and intense physical stress. They have also suggested that besides being a storage for energy, fat tissues help protect the body from severe metabolic impairments that are life-threatening. Based on evidence, it has been speculated that fat tissues serve as a sink for toxins and lipids, protecting the body from their harmful effects. It is also now known that fat tissues serve as a manufacturing site for hormones, particularly the female hormone estrogen. Under certain conditions, this last property of fat tissues can cause disorders and disease in women and men. We'll cover this topic later on.

Finally, the body may be programmed to protect itself from the adverse effects of chronic overfeeding or underfeeding by regulating the rate of fat breakdown or fat gain accordingly. This control mechanism is influenced by one factor: the efficiency with which the body utilizes fat for energy. The greater the body's ability to utilize fat and energy, the lower the levels of plasma and liver lipids will be, and the more likely fat will be mobilized for energy. On the other hand, if the body's ability to utilize fat for energy is diminished, the more likely it is that lipids and cholesterol will accumulate, and fat tissues will tend to enlarge and be more resistant to fat-burning.

High fat utilization and high energy turnover are the key principles for effective fat loss. Let's see how increased fat utilization and high energy turnover can help eliminate the metabolic problems that initially cause fat gain, such as insulin resistance or high levels of toxicity.

Insulin Resistance

Insulin resistance is a metabolic state caused by the accumulation of lipids and cholesterol in the liver and plasma. Hyperlipidemia and fatty liver are correlated with a decreased capacity of the liver to utilize glucose and fat. When glucose utilization decreases, a state of insulin resistance occurs. The body tries to protect itself from insulin resistance by inducing fat gain in a desperate attempt to clear excesses of fatty acids from the blood, liver, and other tissues. In other words, fat gain protects the body from the accumulation of lipids that cause insulin resistance. Ironically, the opposite is also true. As absurd as it may seem, excessive fat breakdown—in particular, the breakdown of visceral fat—may overwhelm the body, leading to over-accumulation of lipids in the plasma and liver, which then causes a state of insulin resistance. In any case, excessive visceral fat, particularly in the belly and waist, increases the risk for insulin resistance that, as noted, may further inhibit fat loss and promote the formation of stubborn fat.

Insulin promotes fat gain, increasing the net uptake of fatty acids into adipocytes. It is considered to be an antilipolytic (anti-fat-burning) hormone. Indeed, insulin has a profound inhibitory effect on biological processes that induce the breakdown of fat for energy. The many inhibitory mechanisms by which insulin slows or prevents lipolysis aren't fully understood. Nonetheless, following are some of the notable ones.

- Insulin stimulates the enzyme phosphodiesterase 3, which degrades and decreases cellular factor cAMP in fat cells. As we've seen, cAMP is critical for lipolysis, and suppressing cAMP inhibits fat-burning.
- Insulin desensitizes beta-adrenoreceptors by inducing translocation of beta-adrenoreceptors to intracellular space, a process that temporarily reduces lipolytic sensitivity to adrenal hormones.
- Insulin inhibits the fat-burning, hormone-sensitive lipase by enhancing its dephosphorylation.

Toxicity

Besides protecting the body from insulin resistance, fat gain serves as a protection from the accumulation of toxins. This is true for both humans and animals. Some of the deadliest industrial toxins are fat-soluble and are stored in fat tissues of marine and mammalian species. For that matter, most of the toxins we get from animal food are concentrated in the fat of fish, beef, pork, or poultry. These very toxins will most likely find their way to the fat tissue of the human consumer. Fat tissues store harmful toxins to protect vital organs from damage. Any process that detoxifies the body will help eliminate this very reason for fat gain, and therefore will help promote fat loss.

To sum up, fat loss requires the following steps:

1. *Increased fat utilization.*
2. *Increased energy turnover.*
3. *Increased detoxification.*

Let's examine how the above translate into actual fat loss and, in particular, the loss of stubborn fat.

Step 1:
Increased Fat Utilization

Most fat utilization occurs in the cell's mitochondria. The greater the number of mitochondrial enzymes, the more efficient fat utilization will be. Because muscle is the largest mitochondria-containing tissue, muscle composition directly affects fat utilization. Certain muscle fiber types have superior fat-utilizing capabilities compared to other muscle fiber types. By virtue of their large mitochondrial capacity, slow muscle fiber types and super muscle fiber types can metabolize fat more efficiently than fast fiber types.

For increased fat utilization and enhanced fat loss, a special training routine may be required. Incorporating endurance, strength, speed, and explosive exercise all together in special drills will most likely signal the body to increase its ability to intensely perform multiple tasks by developing muscle fibers with superior capabilities and increased capacity to utilize fat for energy.

Step 2:
Increased Energy Turnover

"Energy turnover" describes the overall energy that the body consumes, utilizes, and spends. High energy turnover is a state in which the body's metabolic rate is high (high energy expenditure and high food consumption). When energy turnover is high, utilization of carbs and fat increases, thus preventing the accumulation of lipids in the blood and liver.

This highly energetic state could be established by the incorporation of intense physical training and rest intervals with feeding cycles that deplete and pump the fuel needed to charge and accelerate the metabolic machine.

As previously noted, periodic overeating can help increase the body's metabolic rate, thus helping facilitate a state of high energy turnover. Overeating should be always fully controlled and alternated with periodic undereating to prevent a state of chronic overfeeding that can eventually lead to fat gain.

Finally, high energy turnover can be easily manipulated to further promote weight loss. One way of doing that is by alternating between days of high carbs and low carbs, as well as days of undereating and days of overeating. Doing so will induce temporary states of low insulin impact and negative energy balance, respectively, both of which are necessary for a viable fat-burning process to take place. Meanwhile, the days of overeating with their energy-boosting impact will help protect the body's metabolic rate from falling.

These temporary states of low insulin and negative energy balance in an already highly energized body can accelerate fat loss in a most effective way. The above cycles can be adjusted according to individuals' specific needs. Some may need to incorporate three days of undereating followed by one day of overeating, whereas others may find that one day of undereating followed by one day of overeating is highly effective in promoting fat loss. As a general rule, always attempt to keep the diet as low-glycemic as possible. Also avoid overtraining and be sure to nourish your body properly. Overtraining and insufficient nutrition may cause a metabolic decline and a fat gain rebound.

Step 3:
Increased Detoxification

The most effective way to purge the body of toxins naturally is to fast or undereat. When food consumption is minimized, more energy is shifted toward cleansing. And less food means reduced exposure to dietary toxins.

Be aware that effective detoxification increases the release of toxins into the bloodstream and may cause a temporary elevation of circulating free radicals. Whenever you detox, it is important to nourish and supplement your body with antioxidants to help protect it from the oxidative stress and the harmful effects of released toxins. Antioxidants are naturally found in fruits, vegetables, roots, seeds, nuts, mushrooms, and herbs as well as bran and grain germs. Of utmost importance are plant foods such as broccoli, cauliflower, beets, and parsley, known for their substantial liver-detoxifying properties.

If not removed, toxins may accumulate in the liver, kidneys, joints, and other tissues.

Extreme fat-loss methods, including crash diets, can cause an abrupt increase in blood toxin levels that may overwhelm the body and force it to induce fat gain to desperately reabsorb the released toxins. Gradual fat loss is therefore the best way to avoid over-toxicity and fat gain rebound.

Anything that increases toxicity may inhibit fat loss. Food chemicals, pesticides, plastic derivatives such as from polluted water or food containers, as well as excessive alcohol consumption, and certainly chronic constipation are all factors that contribute to increased toxicity, causing accumulation of harmful substances in fat tissues, some of which are known as hormonal disrupting chemicals (nonylphenols, PCBs, organochloride pesticides). These industrial chemicals have been shown to induce health-shattering, sterilizing, and fattening effects on humans and animals.[7] The growing levels of toxins increase the overall metabolic stress on the body, with sometimes overwhelming effects on the liver, compromising its ability to perform its duties. Symptoms of an overwhelmed liver include insulin resistance, hypertension (high blood pressure), increased estrogenic activity, and stubborn fat gain.

Understanding the biological reasons behind fat gain can be of great practical value for people who want to lose fat and stay lean. However, there are additional biological functions of fat tissue that are worthy of our attention.

Regulation of Body Fat via Set Points

Scientists suggest that body fat is regulated by inherent set points of body fat percentage. These inherent set points are primarily markers of how much fat the body can potentially gain or lose. Under certain circumstances such as with obese individuals, the body fat set point serves as a borderline, protecting the person by suppressing any additional fat gain beyond this specific set point. The higher the set point is, the more fat a person will be able to gain.

Body fat is influenced by insulin sensitivity, with insulin tending to inhibit fat-burning. However, beyond a certain set point of body fat gain, the body will be forced to induce a state of insulin resistance to swiftly suppress any additional fat gain. Apparently beyond a certain set point of fat gain, obesity will lead to diabetes. This is how this process occurs on the cellular level.

When insulin-resistant fat cells resist the insulin inhibitory effect, they break spontaneously, releasing fatty acids to the blood. However, this alleged fat breakdown comes at a price: These fatty acids can't be oxidized for energy because fat utilization is suppressed due to lipid and cholesterol accumulation in the liver and the circulatory system. This will cause further accumulation of fatty acids, and if left untreated can lead to diabetes and cardiovascular disease, both of which are associated with increased rates of mortality.

Frequent and Over-Consumption of Carbs

Frequent carbohydrate snacks and over-consumption of processed carbs have been shown to adversely affect insulin receptor sensitivity, thereby leading to high insulin levels, a condition known as hyperinsulinemia. Chronic insulin stimulation from frequent carb consumption during the day may increase insulin resistance toward the end of the day. Minimizing carb consumption to one meal per day, as well as alternating between days of low carbs and days of moderate carbs, may help stabilize insulin sensitivity and afford effective fat loss.

Fat Loss and Exposure to Cold Temperatures

Fat metabolism can be accelerated by exposure to cold temperatures, a fact that can be manipulated to accelerate fat loss. When exposed to extremely cold temperatures, the body increases its energy expenditure, which translates into body heat. This increase in energy production is mediated by certain peptides called uncoupling proteins, which are found in the inner mitochondrial membranes. Uncoupling proteins generate their actions by transferring anions (negatively charged particles) through mitochondrial membranes, leading to a proton infusion that bypasses energy utilization as adenosine triphosphate (ATP), thus inducing what is considered a waste of energy in the form of heat.

Through their thermogenic actions, uncoupling proteins reduce the cellular level of ATP and thereby create a negative cellular energy balance. This negative energy balance signals the body to increase cellular energy production to compensate for the wasted energy. While the body shifts energy production into an overdrive, the negative energy balance within the cell increases the level of cAMP that inhibits insulin and thus promotes fat loss.

A person can take advantage of uncoupling-protein activity through exposure to cold, such as by taking cold showers. The recommended method is to alternate the water temperature between warm and cold and to finish with a cold rinse. Exposing the body to extreme cold has been used traditionally in Europe and Russia. Rubbing snow on the body and jumping into icy rivers are still considered effective methods of improving circulation and overall health.

For the purpose of losing fat, temporary exposure to extremely cold temperatures increases the actions of uncoupling proteins, thereby increasing body heat as well as the rate of fatty acid mobilization and fat loss. Individuals with heart problems or other medical conditions should consult with their health care practitioner before using the above methods.

Ironically, just the opposite may occur when the body is inherently adapted to cold climates. Some individuals are naturally inclined to have stubborn fat because of a genetic predisposition to cold climates. Inuits, Aleutians, and Native North Americans may possess a genetic code that helps them survive in the cold Arctic climate. Having to survive under such extreme environmental conditions, the body must constantly mobilize fatty acids as fuel for energy and heat. Therefore, people who live in extremely cold climates are genetically more predisposed to a high visceral fat level that constantly mobilizes this necessary flux of fatty acids to the liver to be converted to energy and heat. However, this feature that is so beneficial in an extremely cold environment can be detrimental in warm climate conditions, where high visceral fat is correlated with insulin resistance, diabetes, and obesity.

This assumption is part of an evolutionary theory based on the formation of different human body types via adaptation to different climates. Generally, people who live in warm weather are more inclined and biologically suited to eat plant foods such as vegetables, fruits, and grains and are therefore more insulin-sensitive.

People who live in cold climates fare better by eating flesh and fat but may be inherently inclined to an insulin-resistant metabolic state that permits a constant influx of fatty acids to the liver as fuel to keep the body warm. It is currently fashionable to present Inuits as paragons of health. Unfortunately, as healthy as they may be in their native environment, they suffer from myriad blood sugar and vascular problems as soon as they begin to follow a typical Western diet.

People who are genetically predisposed to survive well in cold weather may have a tendency for insulin resistance and stubborn fat gain. Inuits, some Native Americans, and perhaps even some Latino people of part Indian and part Spanish descent may need a special modified diet based on low-glycemic meals. They also need to be physically active, thus creating a state of increased energy expenditure that mimics the way their bodies are originally designed to function. Periodic undereating and a steady exercise routine incorporating both endurance exercise and resistance are highly recommended.

Stress and Stubborn Fat

Fat loss is a process that depends almost exclusively on adrenal hormone actions. Apparently, it is the balance between beta and alpha adrenoreceptors that dictates whether fat tissue is responsive to fat-burning or not. Generally, a fat tissue with high affinity for beta receptors is more reactive to adrenaline's fat-burning effect than a fat tissue with a high affinity for alpha receptors. In fact, alpha-2 receptors inhibit fat-burning because of their suppressive effect on the enzyme adenylate cyclase and its related cellular factor, cAMP. Again, the following may seem a bit technical, but the issue here is critically important for understanding the real contributing factors behind fat loss.

The binding of adrenal hormones to their various receptors creates distinctly different effects on stress reactions and overall fat-burning. Adrenal binding to beta-2 receptors activates an intramembrane G protein that stimulates the synthesis of cellular factor cAMP, which induces fat-burning by activating hormone-sensitive lipase. Fat-tissue breakdown requires the actions of hormone-sensitive lipase; otherwise, fat-burning will be inhibited. In contrast, the binding of adrenal hormones to alpha-2 receptors activates intramembrane GI, which has an inhibitory effect on cAMP, thus suppressing hormone-sensitive lipase and overall fat-burning. There are also alpha-1 and beta-3 adrenoreceptors. The alpha-1 adrenoreceptor may mediate muscle-fueling during physical activity.

Beta-3 receptors are the subject of current research because of their direct response to the neurotransmitter acetylcholine, which facilitates muscle contraction. Beta-3 receptors are considered fat-burning stimulators. Adrenal hormones (catecholamines) are released largely as a fight-or-flight response to stress. The effects of stress on fat-burning are quite complex. Stress causes a release of fatty acids and glucose from the liver and the adipose tissues. In skeletal muscles, stress-related adrenal stimulation causes the breakdown of glycogen reserves to provide immediate fuel for swift reactions. During stress, adrenal hormones accelerate the heart rate to increase blood flow. They also enhance breathing and overall detoxification by relaxing blood vessels in the nasal passages and gastrointestinal tract. In the short run, adrenal hormones help the body react to immediate danger or stress by facilitating fat-burning for immediate fuel utilization, enhancing oxygenation, and eliminating toxins. When chronically stimulated, however, adrenal hormones have other metabolic effects that appear contradictory and confusing.

All adrenoreceptors compete for the same adrenal hormones. Because the ratio of beta- to alpha-adrenoreceptors dictates stimulatory or inhibitory adrenal effects, both stimulatory and inhibitory adrenal actions may serve different biological purposes. A high affinity of a tissue for the inhibitory effect of alpha-2 adrenoreceptors may be part of a biological defense mechanism that protects the body against stress-related adrenal over-excitatory impact.

Over-excitatory impact, which occurs during chronic stress or constant exposure to danger, can lead to chronic anxiety, adrenal exhaustion, and an overall metabolic breakdown. If insufficient rest is combined with chronic stress, the result may be formation of tissues that resist adrenal stimulation, such as with stubborn fat, which typically expresses a high ratio of alpha- to beta-adrenoreceptors and is less responsive to adrenal stimulation. Sufficient rest, sufficient sleep, avoiding overtraining, and utilizing relaxation methods can help manage stress and protect against adrenal exhaustion.

Let stress work for you rather than against you. Short-term, controlled exposure to stress is stimulatory and most effective toward fat loss, whereas chronic or prolonged stress may cause adverse effects. In other words, short, intense workout sessions with sufficient rest yield better results than do protracted workout routines six or seven days a week.

The body adapts to the type of stimulation it experiences most frequently. It follows, then, that the body may adapt to chronic stress by reversing tissue sensitivity to adrenostimulatory reactions to stress, thereby protecting the body from over-excitatory impact and total exhaustion. Adaptation to chronic stress may come at the price of rendering fat tissues less responsive.

Lipolysis: The Chemistry of Fat-Burning

Lipolysis is a process that involves the release and mobilization of fatty acids from adipose tissue to be utilized as fuel. In this simple process, fatty acids attached to glycerol are hydrolytically removed. Fatty acids, in addition to being mobilized for fuel, act as precursors for the synthesis of ketone bodies, such as during prolonged starvation. In addition to breaking fat-storing tissues, lipolysis occurs in muscle tissue and in the liver, where small amounts of fatty acids are stored to produce energy.

The process of lipolysis (or fat-burning) occurs in three stages:

1. Hormonal stimulation.
2. Mobilization of fatty acids to the mitochondria for energy utilization.
3. Fat and energy metabolites signal the body whether to keep mobilizing fat for energy or stop the fat-burning process.

Low-Carb Ketogenic Diets

Ketogenic diets are based on extreme carb deprivation. The motivating idea behind these diets is to create a metabolic state in which the body is forced to increase production of fat metabolites known as ketone bodies (due to an increased demand for fatty acid oxidation) as a substitute for carb fuel. In early stages of the diet, the lack of dietary carbs and low insulin increases the mobilization of fatty acids for fuel and increases liver synthesis of ketone bodies in the form of acetoacetate, 3-hydroxybutyrate, and acetone. Ketones serve as fuel for peripheral tissue, and their formation spares protein breakdown. Promoters of ketogenic diets promise maximum fat loss when ketosis is induced.

What is seemingly great in theory, however, does not always work in reality, and ketogenic diets are doomed to fail from the get-go. People who experience extreme prolonged carb restriction reach a stagnation point or plateau beyond which they cannot lose any more body fat. Moreover, ketogenic diets, if done chronically, may lead to a total metabolic decline, causing dieters to gain back all the weight they initially lost, but this time with a higher percentage of body fat. The reason why ketogenic diets fail is simple: During ketosis, blood pH declines as the body's acidity rises. Desperate to counteract the acidifying effect of ketosis, the body will secrete insulin, which will inhibit lipolysis and thus suppress ketosis, rendering the body resistant to fat-burning. Ketone bodies are acid fat metabolites. The body tries to get rid of them through the lungs and the kidneys, via exhalation and the urine, respectively. However, as noted previously, when the body reaches ketosis, it secretes insulin as a desperate attempt to prevent further acidosis. Insulin inhibits lipolysis and therefore decreases mobilization of fatty acids to the liver. This way, fat loss is suppressed, the synthesis of the liver's ketone bodies decreases, and the body's pH rises. To briefly sum it up, advanced ketosis inhibits fat loss and increases insulin levels, and thus the ketogenic diet's quest of reaching ketosis clearly fails to induce fat loss.

Another problem with ketogenic diets is their suppressing effect on the body's metabolic rate. Chronic extreme carb restrictions adversely reduce cellular adenosine triphosphate, thus impairing thyroid hormone activation—that is, conversion of T4 to the active form, T3. Low thyroid activity is associated with impaired muscle fuel utilization, lack of strength, sensitivity to cold, and fat gain.

Low-carb ketogenic diets are very popular these days. People who suffer from insulin resistance may benefit from low-carb diets adjusted to their individual needs. Nevertheless, the attempt to reach a metabolic state of ketosis for losing fat (such as with extreme high-fat, no-carb diets) is misleading, ill-advised, and counter-effective.

Fat-Burning Hormones

Adrenal hormones are the most important stimulators of lipolysis. Fat cells have three different beta-adrenoreceptors (beta-1, -2, and -3) and alpha-2 adrenoreceptors. While beta-2 and beta-3 receptors stimulate fat burning, alpha-2 and beta-1 receptors may actually inhibit fat breakdown. Adrenal hormones stimulate fat-burning or lipolysis by binding to beta receptors that are coupled to G-sensitive protein. Activated G protein catalyzes the formation of cAMP. cAMP activates protein kinase A, which then finally phosphorylates and activates hormone-sensitive lipase, thus inducing lipolysis. Other fat-burning hormones that also have a cAMP lipolytic effect on fat cells are the thyroid-stimulating hormone and glucagon, hunger-related cholecystokinin, and parathyroid hormone—all stimulators of lipolysis via cAMP activation, but their effects are minor compared to those of the adrenal hormones. The main physiological factors that increase lipolysis are fasting, undereating, and exercise. Each of these physiological factors involves the stimulatory effect of adrenal hormones and the activation of cellular factor cAMP.

Practical Tips for Eliminating the Reasons for Fat to Accumulate

- Establishing temporary states of negative energy balance (when more energy is spent than is consumed) through periodic undereating and exercise will help eliminate the reason for fat to serve as storage for energy and instead will force it to break down as fuel for energy.
- Cleansing the body through periodic fasting or undereating with detoxifying foods and herbs will help neutralize and remove toxins, thus eliminating the reason for fat to serve as a storage for toxins.

- Natural methods that increase the body's capacity to utilize fat for energy, such as incorporating strength, speed, and endurance drills in workout routines, will help protect the body against accumulation of serum lipids, preventing insulin resistance and fat gain.
- Avoiding consumption of hormonal-disrupting substances such as petroleum-based food chemicals, pesticides, fertilizers, and plasticizers, as well as estrogen-promoting foods and herbs and alcohol, will help prevent hormonal disorders, over-estrogenic activity, loss of virility, and stubborn fat gain in men and women.
- Avoiding chronic calorie restrictions and crash diets will help prevent a total metabolic decline and a fat gain rebound.
- Avoiding ketogenic diets that involve extreme chronic carb restrictions can help avoid low thyroid, sluggish metabolism, and a metabolic resistance to fat loss.
- Body exposure to extreme cold temperatures such as by taking cold showers or swimming in cold water will promote a thermogenic effect (via uncoupling proteins) that, besides increasing body heat, will increase the rate of fatty acid mobilization for energy and overall fat loss.
- Avoid chronic stress (such as from overtraining combined with chronic stress or lack of rest) and insufficient nutrition to prevent adrenal exhaustion with a decreased responsiveness to fat-burning stimulation and a resultant sluggish metabolism and fat gain.

PART IV

Muscle Gain and Fat
Loss Conclusions

CHAPTER 10

Insulin's Essential Role
in Muscle Gain and Fat Loss

I nsulin is the most misunderstood hormone and probably the most controversial one. Due to the increased popularity of current low-carb diets, there is an ever-growing number of people with "carb phobias" who view insulin as a hormone that promotes fat gain and disease. Hyper-insulinemia or over-spiking of insulin has indeed been regarded as the main culprit for the current epidemic of weight gain, obesity, and certainly diabetes. But what many people fail to realize is that, despite its reputation as a fat-loss inhibitor, insulin's biological functions are critically important for muscle gain as well as for fat loss. Nowadays, many people choose to follow extreme low-carb diets, hoping to minimize insulin activity and lose weight by chronically restricting carbs to a minimum intake. Low-carb diets, with their extreme restrictions, often lead to frustration rather than long-term leanness. Let's first examine the unique and sometimes tricky ways in which insulin acts or interferes with the actions of other hormones, and how it affects muscle gain and fat loss.

Insulin and IGF1

Insulin plays a critical role in promoting the actions of insulin-like growth factor 1 (IGF1), which facilitates swift anabolic actions in the muscle. Insulin and IGF1 are peptide hormones with similar molecular structures. Both IGF1 and insulin are potent anabolic agents that can inhibit breakdown of muscle protein while promoting amino acids uptake, DNA synthesis, and muscle mass gain. Nonetheless, insulin tends to inhibit fat loss, whereas IGF1 does the opposite.

In addition to the homology between insulin and IGF1, a collaborative mechanism exists between these two hormones. Metabolically, insulin promotes IGF1 actions in a similar way that a big brother takes care of his younger sibling. To be fully effective, IGF1 requires insulin interference. In fact, insulin stimulates IGF1 secretion by the liver. Additionally, growth hormone, which stimulates IGF1, is largely ineffective without the influence of insulin, which may explain why diabetes is often associated with low levels of IGF1 and depressed growth. Insulin and IGF1 work together, however, in a way that may seem contradictory or confusing. In the short run, serum IGF1 levels increase when insulin levels decrease. Moreover, IGF1 receptors in muscle cells increase significantly during periodic fasting.

Lack of food and low insulin levels most likely force the body to increase the number of IGF1 receptors in muscles as compensation in order to potentially maximize performance under extreme conditions of minimal food intake. Researchers believe that the ratio of IGF1 receptors to insulin could be an indicator of metabolic efficiency. Obese people often demonstrate a lower ratio of GH and IGF1 to insulin. However, as mentioned previously, both GH and IGF1 actions can be fully effective only when insulin levels increase, such as when carbs are consumed.

To take full advantage of this complicated way in which insulin affects IGF1, try incorporating periodic fasting or undereating, combined with exercise as recommended, followed by post-exercise recovery meals that include protein and carbs. "Training on empty" enhances the signal to increase both growth hormone and IGF1 receptors in the muscles. Then, to finalize the actual actions of growth hormone and IGF1, one should have recovery meals immediately after exercise that include protein and carbs. It's also critically important to nourish the body with main meals that contain all essential nutrients and sufficient amounts of fuel.

Thus in order to facilitate and not compromise the anabolic actions of growth hormone and IGF1, both of which profoundly affect muscle growth and fat loss, one should avoid chronic carb restrictions. Incorporating periodic cycles of undereating and exercise followed by post-exercise recovery meals may be the best way to initially promote growth hormone and IGF1 and then finalize their actual anabolic actions.

Insulin and the Thyroid Hormones

Insulin enhances thyroid activity in various ways. Thyroid hormones, particularly T3, play a critical role in energy utilization and body heat regulation. The thyroid hormones' actions are also vitally important for potency, cognitive functions, strength, and a healthy body composition. Low thyroid activity is associated with a lowered metabolism as well as decreased mental and physical capacity. Thyroid activity is determined by cellular energy levels, and when cellular energy is low, levels of ATP decrease and the conversion of T4 to its active T3 form is compromised. Insulin, which primarily increases cellular energy and ATP levels, is necessary for fully activating the thyroid hormone T3.

Thyroid hormone activity is also enhanced by the enzyme nitric oxide synthase, which again is stimulated by insulin. This enzyme is responsible for the production of nitric oxide, which plays an important role in the regulation of vasodilation, sexual performance, and growth. Therefore, insulin sensitivity and carb ingestion are essential for proper thyroid functioning, thereby supporting virility, muscularity, and a healthy metabolism.

Suppression of insulin due to chronic carb restriction may cause chronic elevation of the thyroid-stimulating hormone; when this is overexpressed it may cause desensitization of the thyroid's receptors, a condition that further suppresses thyroid hormone actions leading to a sluggish metabolism. And as if this weren't bad enough, chronically high levels of thyroid-stimulating hormone are associated with increased levels of prolactin, the female lactation hormone. In men, elevated prolactin can be detrimental, with a profound feminization effect on the body.

Insulin's actions are also necessary for thyroid hormone synthesis, an intense biochemical process that involves iodinization via brutal oxidative reactions catalyzed by the energy molecule NADPH. The latter is a product of glucose metabolism in the so-called "pentose phosphate pathway" (which is an essential metabolic process derived from insulin-dependent glucose utilization). Though not a steroid, the thyroid hormones have a steroid-like activity, mediating the actions of other anabolic steroids.

This leads to the following conclusions:

- Insulin interference is critical for effective thyroid hormone activity, thereby potentially enhancing muscular development and fat loss.
- Chronic carb and calorie restrictions may impair thyroid function and overall metabolism.
- Insulin sensitivity is paramount for thyroid hormone synthesis.
- Insulin supports anabolic activity via enhancement of the thyroid and steroid hormones.

In summary, by supporting thyroid hormone actions, insulin proves to be a fat-burning enhancer and growth promoter.

Insulin and the Pentose Phosphate Pathway

The pentose phosphate pathway is one of the most critical metabolic pathways in the body, responsible for the production of DNA, RNA, and energy molecules, as well as immuno- and neuro-protective compounds, to name some of its critical functions. This important pathway is totally insulin-dependent. It utilizes glucose for various metabolic functions that affect muscle gain and fat loss. Impaired glucose utilization due to insulin resistance or the accumulation of serum lipids will adversely affect the pentose phosphate pathway, with potentially devastating effects on the body's metabolism.

The pentose phosphate pathway is primarily an anabolic pathway. It utilizes glucose to synthesize the five-carbon-sugar pentose, which plays an essential role in cell membrane, nucleic acid, and steroid hormone biosynthesis. The pentose phosphate pathway is responsible for the utilization of the essential energy molecule NADPH, required for the synthesis of cell nucleus material, including DNA and RNA. This energy molecule is also vital for enhancement of the body's self-defense against DNA damage, as well as protection from oxidant radicals and toxins. NADPH is involved in the recycling of the body's most powerful immune protector—the antioxidant peptide glutathione. The cellular level of unbound (recycled) glutathione serves as a marker for health: the higher the cellular level of unbound glutathione, the more formidable the body's defenses against oxidative stress, disease, and aging.

Glutathione enzymes are responsible for protecting nucleic acids, DNA and RNA from damage, a fact that is of utmost importance because it directly relates to cancer prevention and anti-aging. The importance of the pentose phosphate pathway is often overlooked. Biologically, it serves critical purposes, including the oxidation of glucose to energy. Primary functions include the following:

- Generate the energy molecule NADPH for steroid hormone biosynthesis, as well as to facilitate antioxidant reactions.
- Provide ribose 5 phosphate for the synthesis of nucleotides and the nucleic acids DNA and RNA.
- Regenerate glucose from pentose.

Certain organs such as the liver, adipose tissue, and the adrenal cortex contain high levels of pentose phosphate pathway enzymes. In fact, thirty percent of glucose oxidation in the liver occurs via this biological mechanism.

Again, insulin sensitivity is required for proper glucose utilization and the full activation of its related pentose phosphate pathway. Any intervention in this process may adversely affect the body's ability to handle oxidative stress such as from intense prolonged exercise. As noted previously, through its mediating actions, insulin helps protect the body from genetic damage, thus enhancing immunity and promoting an ongoing anti-aging effect.

Methods that have been shown to help protect against insulin resistance include daily detoxification, minimizing carb consumption to no more than one meal per day, and minimizing simple sugar intake. These are all critical steps that can potentially enhance glucose utilization and effectively support the pentose phosphate pathway. The foods richest in pentose and related enzymes are legumes, particularly mung beans. Interestingly, mung beans were found to increase fertility in chickens, compared to grains or other legume feed. Animal foods, especially meat and liver, are abundant in dietary pentose, which initially stimulates this pathway activity.

As long as the body is insulin-sensitive and sufficiently nourished, it will effectively utilize glucose while sustaining the integrity of the pentose phosphate pathway.

However, prolonged restrictions of carbs and calories may shut down the pentose phosphate pathway, forcing it to produce energy (rather than carrying out its primary functions) in order to compensate for the lack of energy that results from carb and calorie restrictions. All that said, frequent over-consumption of carbs may be as bad as carb restriction, and sometimes worse. Eating too many carb-containing meals during the day may lead to insulin insensitivity, a condition that adversely affects the pentose phosphate pathway and all its beneficial actions.

CHAPTER 11

The Single Overriding Biological Principles of Muscle Gain and Fat Loss

Muscle gain and fat loss are compelling subjects that are pertinent to almost every aspect of life. In spite of the overwhelmingly complex and sometimes contradictory information that we receive, from numerous scientific studies and anecdotal cases, the biological mechanisms that induce muscle gain and fat loss are quite simple.

The purpose of this book is to shed new light on the distinct ways in which muscle and fat tissues operate and to assist people in making responsible decisions about how to effectively improve their body composition and overall performance. As controversial as it may seem, all the information available on muscle gain and fat loss eventually leads to the conclusion that there is indeed a single overriding biological principle that governs whether or not muscle gain and fat loss will occur. The benefits of understanding this principle go far beyond just gaining muscle and/or losing fat. Following this principle can help improve all performance capabilities and enhance all metabolic functions.

The biological principle of muscle gain and fat loss is based on one single factor. The body tends to develop or degrade a tissue according to its particular level of functionality. It is well known that muscle development depends on muscle activity. For that matter, the more functional the muscle is, the more likely it will adapt and develop. Incorporating strength, speed, and endurance exercise through a steady training routine will trigger inherent adaptation mechanisms to improve fiber composition as well as neurological wiring and fueling and thus develop muscles with superior performance and metabolic capabilities.

The same principles apply to fat tissues. Give fat tissue a biological reason to function, and it will increase in size. The four major biological functions of fat tissues are (1) energy storage, (2) toxin storage, (3) protection against insulin resistance, and (4) protection against hormonal imbalance. Eliminating the functions of fat tissue will also eliminate the reasons for its accumulation.

Maintaining a high metabolic rate through exercise and sufficient nutrition, detoxifying through periodic fasting or undereating (including detoxifying food, herbs, and perhaps supplements), maintaining insulin sensitivity through exercise, and minimizing the glycemic index and the frequency of carb meals per day can all be most effective steps in taking away some of the predominant reasons for fat to accumulate. Nevertheless, as noted previously, it's important to avoid crash or starvation diets and refrain from ingesting chemicals that cause hormonal imbalance and fat gain. Stay away from synthetic hormones, pesticides, herbicides, plasticizers, and other petroleum-based chemicals that are estrogen mimickers, all of which have been shown to interrupt the body's hormonal balance, causing fat gain including stubborn fat, metabolic disorders, and cancer. Fat tissues have the capacity to convert androgens to estrogens, a feature that may have played an evolutionary role in regulating estrogen levels in women as well as balancing androgen levels in adult males. Nevertheless, due to the ever-growing onslaught of industrial estrogenic chemicals on our bodies, what initially started as a primal defensive-balancing mechanism in fat tissues has turned now into an adverse and life-threatening process that elevates estrogen to pathological levels in men and women.

Maximize Muscle Functions
While Minimizing Fat Functions

As simple as it may seem, this principle applies to a vast complex of metabolic activities that dictate whether muscle gain or fat loss will occur. It makes sense and translates to actual muscular development and fat loss. By incorporating practical methods that maximize muscle functionality while minimizing the functions of fat tissues, one will be able to improve muscle composition and lean down while taking advantage of other health benefits, including increased insulin sensitivity, improved hormonal balance, improved lipids profile (with lower cholesterol), and superior capacity to utilize carbs and fat for energy.

The idea is quite revolutionary that both muscle and fat tissue serve biological purposes in addition to their traditional functions as a vehicle for motion or storage for energy. The viability of this concept is boosted by the fact that both muscle and fat tissues inherently affect each other's functions. For instance, a highly developed muscle with superior capacity to utilize fat and carbs for energy will help reduce serum lipids and cholesterol while protecting against insulin resistance. And for that matter, this well-developed muscle will help promote fat loss by taking away some of the very biological functions that give fat tissues reasons to exist. On the other hand, excessive accumulation of body fat will most likely antagonize muscular development due to its association with hormonal imbalance and a sluggish metabolism. Fat gain and heavier body weight may compromise muscle functionality, decreasing speed and capacity to resist fatigue; furthermore, excessive fat gain has been correlated with elevated estrogen levels, which adversely affects muscularity.

By following this single solid biological principle, you can enjoy numerous life benefits. The dramatic result will be the development of a leaner, more powerful body with well-defined and superior metabolic capabilities.

The mechanism to improve body performance is already within you. Take advantage of it to transform yourself. Become a super you.

Final Note

The single biological principle of muscle gain and fat loss is based on inherent biological mechanisms that enhance the impact of hormones, increase the efficiency of energy utilization from fat storage, and induce muscular development for superior performance. This principle is real. And for the purpose of clarity, it is important to understand that principles are the constant and unchangeable pillars upon which all practical methods should be based.

All biological principles are correlated with survival. The assumption that survival dictates a hierarchy of life functions might be considered philosophical, yet it is the only assumption that makes sense. Survival appears to be the ultimate reason behind all the numerous biological actions that define life. In times of so much confusion about how to develop muscle and lose fat, it's important to examine the reasons why muscular development and fat loss occur. The goal of this book is to address the purpose behind the actions. Human intelligence and instincts are based on reason and logic. Regardless of whether you believe that life serves a purpose or not, your body operates in a manner that always makes biological sense.

NOTES

1. Desmond Morris, *Man Watching*. United Kingdom: Harper Collins, 1920. Also by the same author: *The Human Zoo* (United Kingdom: Vintage, 1994); *Intimate Behavior* (United Kingdom: Vintage, 1994); and *Human Sexes: The Natural History of Man and Woman* (New York: St. Martin's Press, 1998).

2. *Lancet* 365:1978–1980 (2005).

3. Weddle, D.L., Tithoff, P., Williams, M., and Schuller, H.M. 2001. ß-Adrenergic growth regulation of human cancer cell lines derived from pancreatic ductal carcinomas. *Carcinogenesis* 3:473–479.

4. Giurisato, E., Dalla Libera, L., Ravara, B., Massimino M.L., and Cantini, M. (1998). Myo-D positive cells overcome fibroblasts in primary muscle cultures grown in the presence of a 50-10 kDa cytokind secreted by macrophages. *Basic Appl Myol* 8(5):381–388.

5. Brodsky, I.G., Suzara, D., Furman, M., Goldspink, P., Ford, G.C., Sreekumaran Nair, K., Kukowski, J., and Bedno, S. 2004. Proteasome production in human muscle during nutritional inhibition of myofibrillar protein degradation. *Metabolism* 53(3):340–347.

6. National Center for Health Statistics. Centers for Disease Control and Prevention. "Obesity Still a Major Problem." Press release, April 14, 2006.

   http://www.cdc.gov/nchs/pressroom/06Facts/obesity03_04.htm
   http://www.cdc.gov/nchs/pressroom/06Facts/obesity03_04.htm

7. Colburn, T., Dumanoski, D., and Peterson Myers, J. *Our Stolen Future*. New York: Plume/Penguin Books, 1996.

   Morse, D.C., Koeter, H.B.W.M., van Prooijen, A.E.S., and Brouwer A. 1992. Interference of polychlorinated biphenyls in thyroid hormone metabolism: possible neurotoxic consequences in fetal and neonatal rats. *Chemosphere* 25 (1, 2):165–168.

   Wolff, M.S., Toniolo, P.G., Lee, E.W., Rivera, M., and Dubin, N. 1993. Blood levels of organochlorine residues and risk of breast cancer. *J Natl Cancer Inst* 85(8):648–652.

REFERENCES

Alderton, W., Cooper, C., and Knowles, R. 2001. Nitric oxide synthases: Structure, function and inhibition. *Biochem. J.* 357:593–615.

Andriamampandry, M., Bnouham, M., Michard, D., Gutbier, G., LeMaho, Y., and Candriamampandry, L. 1996. Food deprivation modifies fatty acid partitioning and beta-oxidation capacity in rat liver. *J. Nutr.* 126(8):2020–2027.

Anson, R., Guo, Z., deCabo, R., Iyun, T., Rios, M., Hagepanos, A., Ingram, D., Lane, M., and Mattson, M. 2003. Intermittent fasting dissociates beneficial effects of dietary restriction on glucose metabolism and neuronal resistance to injury from calorie intake. *Proc. Natl. Acad. Sci.* 100(10):6216–6220.

Arner, P. 2001. Regional differences in protein production by human adipose tissue. *Biochem. Soc. Trans.* 29:72–75.

Beck, B., Stricker-Krongrad, A., Burlet, A., Nicolas, J., and Burlet, C. 1992. Specific hypothalamic neuropeptide Y variation with diet parameters in rats with food choice. *Neuroreport* 3(7):571–574.

Benthem, L., van der Leest, J., Steffens, A., and Zijlstra, W. 1995. Metabolic and hormonal responses to adrenoreceptor antagonists in 48-hour-starved exercising rats. *Metabolism* 44(10):1332–1339.

Bereket, A., Wilson, T., Kolasa, A., Fan, J., and Lang, C. 1996. Regulation of the insulin-like growth factor system by acute acidosis. *Endocrinology* 137(6):2238–2245.

Bergstrom, J., Hermansen, L., Hultman, E., and Saltin, B. 1967. Diet, muscle glycogen and physical performance. *Acta Physiol. Scand.* 71:140–150.

Bergstrom, S. 1982. The prostaglandins: From the laboratory to the clinic. Nobel lecture, 8 December. Karolinska Institutet: Stockholm, Sweden.

Blaukat, A., and Dikic, I. 2001. Activation of sphingosine kinase by the bradykinin B2 receptor and its implication in regulation of the ERK/MAP kinase pathway. *Biol. Chem.* 382:135–139.

Bogardus, C., LaGrange, B., Horton, E., and Sims, E. 1981. Comparison of carbohydrate-containing and carbohydrate-restricted hypocaloric diets in the treatment of obesity. Endurance and metabolic fuel homeostasis during strenuous exercise. *Am. J. Clin. Invest.* 68(2):399–404.

Brodsky, I.G., Suzara, D., Furman, M., Goldspink, P., Ford, G.C., Sreekumaran Nair, K., Kukowski, J., and Bedno, S. 2004. Proteasome production in human muscle during nutritional inhibition of myofibrillar protein degradation. *Metabolism* 53(3):340–347.

Brun, S., Carmona, C., Mampel, T., Vinas, O., Giralt, M., Iglesias, R., and Villarroya, F. 1999. Uncoupling protein-3 gene expression in skeletal muscle during development is regulated by nutritional factors that alter circulating non-esterified fatty acids. *FEBS Lett.* 453(1–2):205–209.

Butler, J. 2001. Biochemical tests of growth hormone status in short children. *Ann. Clin. Biochem.* 38:1–2.

Cai, A., Widdowson, P., Harrold, J., Wilson, S., Buckingham, R., Arch, J., Tadayyon, M., Clapham, J., Wilding, J., and Williams, G. 1999. Hypothalamic orexin expression: Modulation by blood glucose and feeding. *Diabetes* 48(11):2132–2137.

Cakir, Y., Plummer, H., Tithof, P., and Schuller, H. 2002. Beta-adrenergic and arachidonic acid-mediated growth regulation of human breast cancer cell lines. *Int. J. Oncol.* 21:153–157.

Chan, C., DeLeo, D., Joseph, J., McQuaid, T., Ha, X-F, Xu, F., Tsushima, R., Pennefather, P., Salapatek, A., and Wheeler, M. 2002. Increased uncoupling protein-2 levels in b-cells are associated with impaired glucose-stimulated insulin secretion. *PNAS* 99(14):9392–9397.

Chang, J., and Liu, L-Z. 2001. Peroxisome proliferator-activated receptor agonists prevent 25-OH-cholesterol induced c-jun activation and cell death. *Pharmacology* 1:10.

Chaudhuri, A., and Izzo, J. 2000. Insulin resistance and hypertension in the absence of subcutaneous fat. *Rev. Cardiovasc. Med.* 1(2):120–124.

Clapham, J.C., Arch, J.R., Chapman, H., Haynes, A., Lister, C., Moore, G.B., Piercy, V., Carter, S.A., Lehner, I., Smith, S.A., Beeley, L.J., Godden, R.J., Herrity, N., Skehel, M., Changani, K.K., Hockings, P.D., Reid, D.G., Squires, S.M., Hatcher, J., Trail, B., Latcham, J., Rastan, S., Harper, A.J., Cadenas, S., Buckingham, J.A., Brand, M.D., Abuin, A. 2000. Mice overexpressing human uncoupling protein-3 in skeletal muscle are hyperphagic and lean. *Nature.* Jul 27;406(6794):415–418. PMID: 10935638 [PubMed - indexed for MEDLINE]

Clark, M.G., Rattigan, S., Colquboun, E.Q. 1991. Hypertension in obesity may reflect a homeostatic thermogenic response. *Life Sci.*

48(10):939–947. Review. PMID: 2000025 [PubMed - indexed for MEDLINE]

Clark, N. 1951. *Sports Nutrition Guide Book.* Champaign, IL: Human Kinetics.

Coleman, E. 1991. Carbohydrates: The master fuel. In: *Sports Nutrition for the '90s,* eds. Berning, J.R., and Stenn, S.N. Gaithersburg, MD: Aspen Publishers.

Conlee, R. 1987. Muscle glycogen and exercise endurance: A twenty-year perspective. *Ex. Sport. Sci. Rev.* 15:1–28.

Costill, D.L, Sherman, W., Fink, W., Witten, M., and Miller, M. 1981. The role of dietary carbohydrates in muscle glycogen resynthesis after strenuous running. *Am. J. Clin. Nutr.* 34:1831–1836.

Covasa, M., and Ritter, R.C. 1998. Rats maintained on high-fat diets exhibit reduced satiety in response to CCK and bombesin. *Peptides* 19(8):1407–1415. PMID: 9809656 [PubMed - indexed for MEDLINE]

Deferrari, G., Garibotto, G., Robaudo, C., Saffioti, S., Russo, R., and Sofia, A. 1997. Protein and amino acid metabolism in splanchnic organs in metabolic acidosis. *Miner Electrolyte Metab.* 23(3–6):229–233.

Drin, G., Rousselle, C., Scherrmann, J-M., Rees, A., and Temsamani, J. 2002. Peptide delivery to the brain via adsorptive-mediated endocytosis: Advances with SynB vectors. *AAPS PharmSci.* 4(4):26.

Duan, W., Guo, Z., Jaing, H., Ware, M., Li, X-J., and Mattson, M. 2003. Dietary restriction normalizes glucose metabolism and brain-derived neurotropic factor levels, slows disease progression and increases survival in Huntington mutant mice. *Proc. Natl. Acad. Sci.* 100(5):2911–2916.

Dulloo, A., Jacquet, J., and Girardier, L. 1996. Autoregulation of body composition during weight recovery in humans: The Minnesota Experiment revisited. *Int. J. Obes. Relat. Metab. Disord.* 20(5):393–405.

Ehret, A. 1971. *Rational Fasting.* New York: Benedict Lust Publications.

Erasmus, U. 1993. *Fats That Heal, Fats That Kill.* British Columbia, Canada: Alive Books.

Erdkamp, P. 1998. *Hunger and the Sword.* Amsterdam: Gieben.

Erdmann, R. 1987. *The Amino Revolution.* New York: Simon & Schuster.

Evans, S., Lo, H., Ney, D., and Welbourne, T. 1996. Acid-base homeostasis parallels anabolism in surgically stressed rats treated with GH and IGF-I. *Am. J. Physiol.* 270(6):E968–974.

Forslund, A., El-Khoury, A., Olsson, R., Sjödin, A., Hambraeus, L., and Young, V. 1999. Effect of protein intake and physical activity on 24-h pattern and rate of macronutrient utilization. *Am. J. Physiol.* 276(5):E964–976.

Friedman, J.E., Neufer, P.D., and Dohm, G.L. 1991. Regulation of glycogen resynthesis following exercise. Dietary considerations. *Sports Med. Rev.* 11(4):232–243. PMID: 1901662 [PubMed - indexed for MEDLINE]

Garlid, K.D., Jaburek, M., Jezek, P. 2001. Mechanism of uncoupling protein action. *Biochem Soc Trans Rev.* (Pt 6):803–806. PMID: 11709078 [PubMed - indexed for MEDLINE]

Garnsey, P., and Scheidel, W., Eds. 1998. *Cities, Peasants, and Food in Classical Antiquity: Essays in Social and Economic History.* Cambridge, UK: Cambridge University Press.

Giurisato, E., Dalla Libera, L., Ravara, B., Massimino M.L., and Cantini, M. (1998). Myo-D positive cells overcome fibroblasts in primary muscle cultures grown in the presense of a 50-10 kDa cytokind secreted by macrophages. *Basic Appl Myol* 8(5):381–388.

Gregoraszczuk, E.L., and Galas, J. 1998. In Vitro Effect of Triiodothyronine on the Cyclic AMP, Progesterone and Testosterone Level in Porcine Theca, Granulosa and Luteal Cells. *Endocr Regul.* 32(2):93–98. PMID: 10330523 [PubMed - as supplied by publisher]

Hagan, M., Havel, P., Seely, R., Woods, S., Ekhator, N., Baker, D., Hill, K., Wortman, M., Miller, A., Gingerich, R., and Geracioti, T. 1999. Cerebrospinal fluid and plasma leptin measurements: Covariability with dopamine and cortisol in fasting humans. *J. Clin. Endocrinol. Metab.* 84(10):3579–3585.

Hellerstein, M.K, Neese, R.A., Linfoot, P., Christiansen, M., Turner, S., Letscher, A. 1997. Hepatic gluconeogenic fluxes and glycogen turnover during fasting in humans. A stable isotope study. *J Clin Invest.* 100(5):1305–1319. PMID: 9276749 [PubMed - indexed for MEDLINE]

Hocman, G. 1988. Prevention of cancer: Restriction of nutritional energy intake (joules). *Comp. Biochem. Physiol.* 91(2):209–220.

Hornstra, G. 1988. Omega-3 long-chain polyunsaturated fatty acids and health benefits. Prepared by Gerard Hornstra, PhD Med, Professor of Experimental Nutrition, Maastricht University, and Scientific Director of NutriScience BV, a commercial research and consultancy company in the area of novel and functional foods, PO Box 616, 6200 MD Maastricht, Holland tel. +31-43-388 1988; fax: +31-43-388 1530; E-mail: G.Hornstra@NutriScience.NL. Amended and updated version of the English translation of *Oméga-3 et bénéfice santé*, initially published by Catherine Anselmino, Centre d'Etude et d'Information sur les Vitamines, Roche Vitamines France, Neuilly-sur-Seine.

Isidori, A., Massimiliano, C., Strollo, F., Moretti, C., Frajese, G., and Fabbri, A. 1999. Leptin and androgens in male obesity: Evidence for leptin contribution to reduced androgen levels. *J. Clin. Endocrinol. Metab.* 84(10):3673–3680.

Jensen, B. 1993. *Foods That Heal.* Wayne, NJ: Avery Publishing Group.

Jensen, B. 2000. *Guide to Body Chemistry and Nutrition.* Los Angeles: Keats Publishing.

Jiang, X., Russo, I., and Russo, J. 2002. Alternately spliced luteinizing hormone/human chorionic gonadotropin receptor mRNA in human breast epithelial cells. *Int. J. Oncol.* 20:735–738.

Jones, B.S., Yeaman, S.J., Sugden, M.C., Holness, M.J. 1992. Hepatic pyruvate dehydrogenase kinase activities during the starved-to-fed transition. *Biochim Biophys Acta.* Mar 16;1134(2):164–168. PMID: 1554750 [PubMed - indexed for MEDLINE]

Karch, S. 1999. *Herbal Medicine.* Hauppauge, NY: Advanced Research Press.

Katayama, Y., Sakakihara, S., and Maeda, M. 2001. Electrochemical sensing for the determination of activated cyclic AMP-dependent protein kinase. *Anal Sci.* 17(1):17–19. PMID: 11993657 [PubMed - indexed for MEDLINE]

Kersen, S., Seydoux, J., Peters, J., Gonzales, F., Desvergne, B., and Wahli, W. 1999. Peroxisome proliferator-activated receptor alpha mediates the adaptive response to fasting. *J. Clin. Invest.* 103(11):1489–1498.

Lambert, E., Speechly, D., Dennis, S., and Noakes, T. 1994. Enhanced endurance in trained cyclists during moderate-intensity exercise following 2 weeks' adaptation to a high-fat diet. *Eur. J. Appl. Physiol.* 69:387–393.

Lemmens, R., VanDuffel, L., Teuchy, H., and Culic, O. 1996. Regulation of proliferation of LLC-MK2 cells by nucleosides and nucleotides: The role of ectoenzymes. *Biochem. J.* 316:551–557.

Levin, B., and Sullivan, A. 1984. Regulation of thermogenesis in obesity. *Int. J. Obesity* 8(1):159–180.

Ludwig, D., Mazjoub, J., Al-Zahrani, G., Blanco, I., and Roberts, S. 1999. High-glycemic-index foods, overeating, and obesity. *Pediatrics* 103(3):E26.

Marti, A., Berraondo, B., and Martinez, J. 1999. Leptin: Physiological actions. *J. Physiol. Biochem.* 55(1):43–49.

Mellor, H., and Parker, P. 1998. The extended protein kinase C superfamily. *Biochem. J.* 332:281–292.

Mese, H., Sasaki, A., Nakayama, S., Yoshioka, N., Yoshihama, Y., Kishimoto, K., and Matsumura, T. 2002. Prognostic significance of heat-shock protein 27 (HSP27) in patients with oral squamous cell carcinoma. *Oncol. Rep.* 9:341–344.

Minassian, C., Montana, S., and Mithieux, G. 1999. Regulatory role of glucose-6 phosphatase in the repletion of liver glycogen during refeeding in fasted rats. *Biochem. Biophys. Acta.* 1452(2):172–178.

Mondoa, E., and Kiteim, S. 2001. *Sugars That Heal—The New Healing Science of Glyconutrients.* New York: Ballantine.

Morse, D.C., Koeter, H.B.W.M., van Prooijen, A.E.S., and Brouwer A. 1992. Interference of polychlorinated biphenyls in thyroid hormone metabolism: possible neurotoxic consequences in fetal and neonatal rats. *Chemosphere* 25 (1, 2):165–168.

Newby, F., Wilson, L., Thacker, S., and DiGirolamo, M. 1990. Adipocyte lactate production remains elevated during refeeding after fasting. *Am. J. Physiol.* 259(6):E865–871.

Nguyen, L., Karjalainen, A., Milbourne, E., and Bygrave, F. 1998. Permeable analogues of cGMP promote hepatic calcium inflow induced by the synergistic action of glucagon and vasopressin but inhibit that induced by vasopressin alone. *Biochem. J.* 330:877–880.

O'Dea, K., Esler, M., Leonard, P., Stockigt, J.R., and Nestel, P. 1982. Noradrenaline turnover during under- and over-eating in normal-weight subjects. *Metabolism.* (9):896–899. PMID: 7121260 [PubMed - indexed for MEDLINE]

Ogihara, H., Suzuki, T., Nagamachi, Y., Inui, K., and Takata, K. 1999. Peptide transporter in the rat small intestine: ultrastructural localization and the effect of starvation and administration of amino acids. *Histochem J.* 31(3):169–174. PMID: 10421416 [PubMed - indexed for MEDLINE].

Perel, Y., Amrein, L., Dobremez, E., Daniel, J., and Landry, M. 2002. Galanin and galanin receptor expression in neuroblastic tumors: Correlation with their differentiation status. *Br. Canc. J.* 86:117–122.

Phinney, S. 1992. Exercise during and after very-low-calorie dieting. *Am. J. Clin. Nutr.* 56:190S–194S.

Phinney, S.D., Bistrian, B.R, Evans, W.J., Gervino, E., and Blackburn, G.L. 1983. The human metabolic response to chronic ketosis without caloric restriction: preservation of substrate exercise capability with reduced carbohydrate oxidation. *Metabolism* 32(8):769–776.

Phinney, S.D., LaGrange, B.M., O'Connell, M., and Danforth, E., Jr. 1988. Effects of aerobic exercise on energy expenditure and nitrogen balance during very-low-calorie dieting. *Metabolism.* Aug 37(8):758–765. PMID: 3405093 [PubMed - indexed for MEDLINE]

Plata-Salaman, C. 1991. Regulation of hunger and satiety in man. *Dig. Dis.* 9(5):253–268.

Radomski, M., Cross, M., and Buguet, A. 1998. Exercise-induced hyperthermia and hormonal responses to exercise. *Can. J. Physiol. Pharmacol.* 76(5):547–552.

Samec, S., Seydoux, J., and Dulloo, A. 1998. Interorgan signaling between adipose tissue metabolism and skeletal muscle uncoupling protein homologs: Is there a role for circulating free fatty acids? *Diabetes* 47(11):1693–1698.

Samman, S., Lyons-Wall, P., and Farmakalidis, E. Department of Biochemistry, University of Sydney, Australia. 1999. Flavanoids and other phytochemicals in relation to coronary heart disease. In *Antioxidants in Human Health,* Sec. 3, Chap. 15:175–187, edited by T.K. Basu and M.L. Garg. CAB International: N.J.Temple ISBN: 0851993346.

Sandberg, P. 1999. Carbohydrate loading and deploying forces. *Mil. Med.* 164(9):636–642.

Schreihofer, D.A., Parfitt, D.B., and Cameron, J.L. 1993. Suppression of luteinizing hormone secretion during short-term fasting in male rhesus monkeys: the role of metabolic versus stress signals. *Endocrinology* 132(5):1881–1889. PMID: 8477641 [PubMed - indexed for MEDLINE]

Selvais, P.L., Labuche, C., Nguyen, X.N., Ketelslegers, J.M., Denef, J.F., and Maiter, D.M. 1997. Cyclic feeding behaviour and changes in hypothalamic galanin and neuropeptide Y gene expression induced by zinc deficiency in the rat. *J Neuroendocrinol.* 9(1):55–62. PMID: 9023738 [PubMed - indexed for MEDLINE]

Sherman, W., Coastal, D., Fink, W., and Miller, J. 1981. Effect of exercise-diet manipulation on muscle glycogen supercompensation and its subsequent utilization during performance. *Int. J. Sport. Med.* 2:114–118.

Sherman, W. 1983. Carbohydrates, muscle glycogen, and muscle glycogen supercompensation. In *Ergogenic Aids in Sports,* edited by M. Williams. Champagne, IL: Human Kinetics.

Sivitz, W., Fink, B., and Donohue, P. 1999. Fasting and leptin modulate adipose and muscle uncoupling protein: Divergent effects between messenger ribonucleic acid and protein expression. *Endocrinology* 140(4):1511–1519.

Spark, R. 2000. *Sexual Health for Men.* Cambridge, MA: Perseus Books.

Strack, A., Akana, S., Horsley, C., and Dallman, M. 1997. A hypercaloric load induces thermogenesis but inhibits stress responses in the SNS and HPA system. *Am. J. Physiol.* 272(3):R840–848.

Svanberg, E., Jefferson, L., Lundholm, K., and Kimball, S. 1997. Postprandial stimulation of muscle protein synthesis is mediated through translation initiation and is independent of changes in insulin. *APStracts* 4:0030E.

Toppila, J. 1999. (Academic Dissertation) Somatostatin, growth hormone-releasing hormone, galanin and their hypothalamic messenger ribonucleic acids in the regulation of sleep in rats. Institute of Biomedicine, Department of Physiology, University of Helsinki, Finland.

Torrecillas, G., Diez-Marques, M.L., Garcia-Escribano, C., Bosch, R.J., Rodriguez-Puyol, D., and Rodriguez-Puyol, M. 2000. Mechanisms of cGMP-dependent mesangial-cell relaxation: a role for myosin light-chain phosphatase activation. *Biochem J.* 346:217–222.

Wang, J., and Leibowitz, K. 1997. Central insulin inhibits hypothalamic galanin and neuropeptide Y gene expression and peptide release in intact rats. *Brain Res.* 777(1–2):231–236.

Weddle, D.L., Tithoff, P., Williams, M., and Schuller, H.M. 2001. ß-Adrenergic growth regulation of human cancer cell lines derived from pancreatic ductal carcinomas. *Carcinogenesis* 3:473–479.

Welbourne, T., Milford, L., and Carter, P. 1997. The role of growth hormone in substrate utilization. *Baillieres Clin. Endocrinol. Metab.* 11(4):699–700.

Wurtman, J., and Suffes, S. 1997. *Serotonin Solution.* New York: Fawcett Columbine.

Nürnberg, K., Wegner, J., and Ender, K. 1998. Factors influencing fat composition in muscle and adipose tissue of farm animals. Division of Muscle Biology and Growth, Research Institute for Biology of Farm Animals; Wilhelm-Stahl-Allee 2; D-18196 Dummerstorf. *Live. Prod. Sci.* 56:145–156.

Van Voorstl, F., and De Kruijff, Ben. 2000. Review Article: Role of lipids in the translocation of proteins across membranes. Department of Biochemistry of Membranes, CBLE, Institute Biomembranes, Utrecht University, Padualaan 8, 3584 CH Utrecht, The Netherlands. *Biochem. J.* 347:601–612. (Printed in Great Britain)

Vernon, R.G. 2000. Adipocyte studies: systems for investigating effects of growth hormone and other chronically acting hormones. Hannah Research Institute, Ayr KA6 5HL, Scotland, UK. *Biochem. Soc. Trans.* 28:126–131. (Printed in Great Britain)

Wolff, M.S., Toniolo, P.G., Lee, E.W., Rivera, M., and Dubin, N. 1993. Blood levels of organochlorine residues and risk of breast cancer. *J Natl Cancer Inst* 85(8):648–652.

INDEX

ABOUT THE AUTHOR

ORI HOFMEKLER is a modern renaissance man whose formative military experience prompted a life interest in survival science. A graduate of the Bezalel Academy of Art and the Hebrew University in Jerusalem, where he received a degree in Human Science, he is a world-renowned artist whose work has been featured in magazines worldwide. His art books of political satire have been published in the United States and Europe.

As editor-in-chief of *Mind and Muscle Power* magazine, Hofmekler introduced his diet approach to the public to immediate acclaim from readers and professionals. His previous book, *The Warrior Diet,* was first published in 2002 in the United States, France, and Italy, and has been featured in newspapers, magazines, and science journals. A new, revised edition was published in 2007. Hofmekler's 2006 book, *The Anti-Estrogenic Diet,* provides solutions to hormonal-disrupting chemicals in the environment, food, and water. His *Take No Prisoners* newsletter exposes fallacies in the areas of diet and fitness, and presents the true facts about human survival in today's world. For more information, visit warriordiet.com.